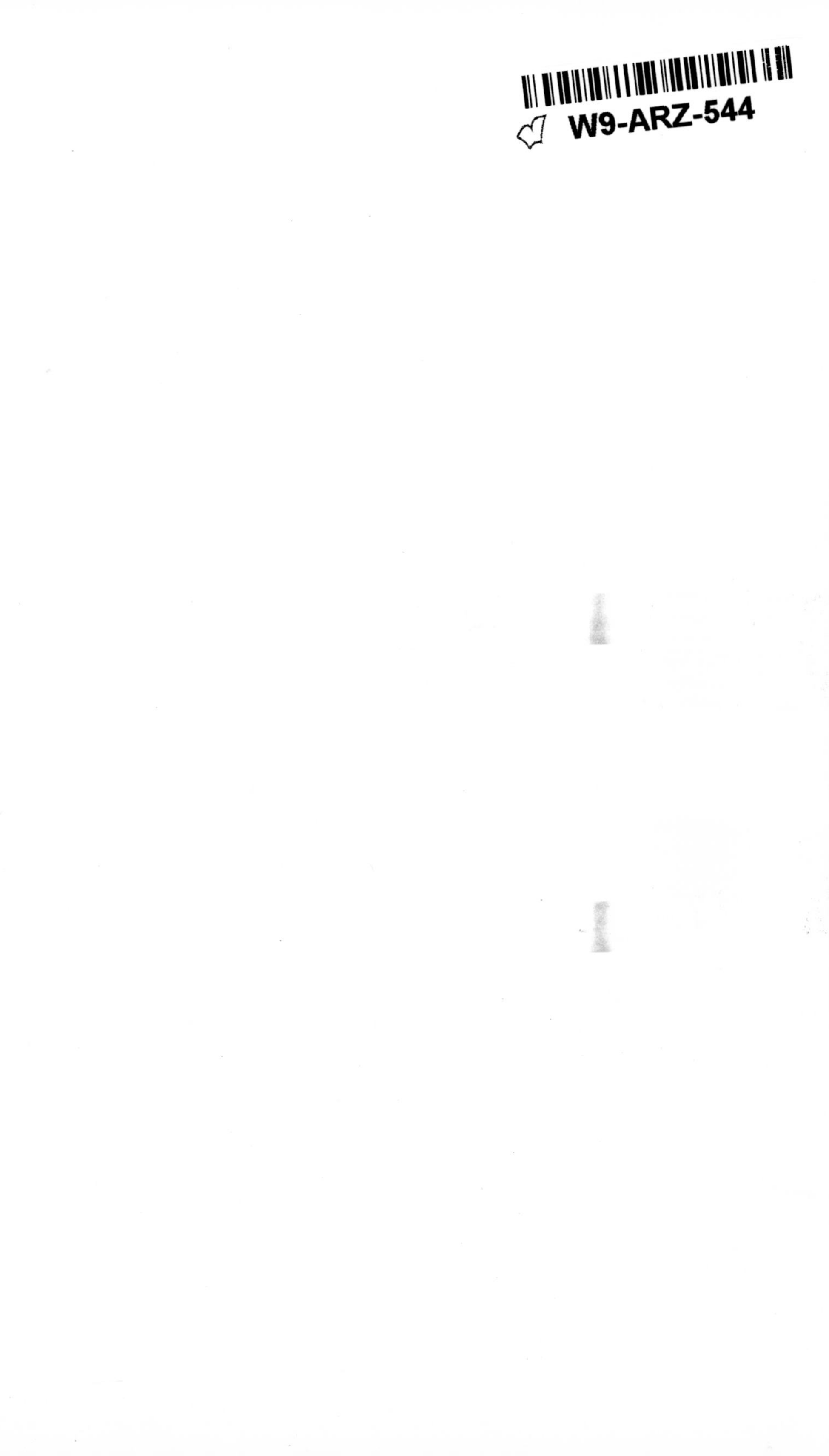

The Rehabilitation Environment

The Rehabilitation Environment

Carroll M. Brodsky
Robert T. Platt
University of California

Lexington Books
D.C. Heath and Company
Lexington, Massachusetts
Toronto

Library of Congress Cataloging in Publication Data

Brodsky, Carroll M
The rehabilitation environment.

Bibliography: p.
1. Psychiatric hospitals–Sociological aspects. 2. Hospitals–Sociological aspects. 3. Rehabilitation centers–Sociological aspects. I. Platt, Robert T., joint author. II. Title.
RC439.B84 362.2′04′25 77-26370
ISBN 0-669-02168-7

Published simultaneously in Canada

Printed in the United States of America

International Standard Book Number: 0-669-02168-7

Library of Congress Catalog Card Number: 77-26370

This book is dedicated to the director and the head nurse of the short-lived rehabilitation unit whose story is chronicled here.

Contents

List of Figures and Tables

Figures

Tables

Preface

During the four years of the study reported in this book, we came to the decision that physicians and medical administrators are unequipped—somewhere in the range from totally to moderately—to design units capable of both approaching humanely the problems of patients and satisfying the needs of staff and students. We were convinced that the problems of medical units, and possibly of other small social organizations, are not primarily people problems but systems problems. Our observations of the birth and death of the rehabilitation unit (and the psychiatric unit that preceded it) suggested some conclusions that might be helpful to administrators and physicians faced with the task of designing a medical system.

We describe in this book some of the events upon which these conclusions are based. Dr. Brodsky is responsible for the theoretical framework within which the events are presented, the elaboration of the implications for planning, and the actual writing of the book. Dr. Brodsky and Dr. Platt collaborated in the analysis and synthesis of the mass of data from the extensive records that were kept and from intensive interviews conducted by them over a one-year period and follow-up interviews held later. A study made in 1973 by Kenneth Payne, an anthropology graduate student working under the supervision of Dr. Brodsky, was an additional and valuable resource.

The project and the book, of course, reflect the work of many persons who contributed in special ways. The important study made by Kenneth Payne has been mentioned. Ruth Ormsby provided invaluable research assistance during the course of the study on the unit, as did Kay Knox during the long and exacting process of evaluating the data and placing it in the context of the available literature. Deborah Gordon and Laura Hill applied research and editorial skills of the highest order during what often seemed the impossible job of shaping a manuscript from the voluminous material available. Mary Ann Esser did the final editing to prepare the manuscript for publication and saw it through the publication process. Karyl Herman lent her endlessly patient and skillful efforts to the typing of the manuscript in its various stages. As usual, thanks seem inadequate to express the authors' gratitude. Even more difficult is the expression of our appreciation for the generous cooperation of the staff and patients of the rehabilitation unit. The crucial importance of their contributions will be evident on every page.

The book began as a study not of a rehabilitation unit but of a psychiatric unit. In 1960, a university medical center decided to establish a program to provide psychiatric services for the private patients of its staff. Because the large neuropsychiatric institute attached to the medical center did not accept private patients, a psychiatrist who referred someone to this facility could not continue to treat the patient; rather, the house staff usually took over the treatment, and the referring psychiatrist never saw the patient again. Both the psychiatrists and other physicians were unhappy with this system and urged the administration to establish a private psychiatric unit. The administration consented.

The time for establishing a new and separate unit was propitious. A large area of the hospital was being remodeled, and one wing was readily converted to psychiatric use. The unit was designed to meet the particular needs of psychiatric patients who, unlike surgical or orthopedic patients, would stay for relatively long periods of time during which they would be ambulatory and dress in street clothes. The unit thus included a dayroom, a kitchen, a laundry room, and a dining room, all intended to provide some of the amenities of home living.

Because no existing unit in the medical center served this particular psychiatric function, an entirely new staff had to be recruited. Those who became the staff hoped to develop a unit with a new spirit, culture, and outlook. They knew that no organization could be formed without the risks that accompany a trial-and-error approach, but the chief medical administrator and the senior author of this study (Dr. Brodsky), the head nurse, and the chief occupational therapist were optimistic. Relatively knowledgeable about interpersonal techniques, they knew the therapeutic and practical value of resolving problems by talking them out.

So, through what was seen as a period of trial and error, the core staff met, talked, and analyzed. They decided that some of their problems were caused by their patients: too many were alcoholics, too many had character disorders, and too many were senile. Other problems, they felt, were caused by members of the staff who for various reasons did not fit: some were too neurotic or had character disorders themselves; some were too hostile; and some simply could not work cooperatively with the others.

As a result of this process of soul-searching, studying, and blaming, the core staff began to be more selective in accepting patients for treatment. They also applied sufficient pressure that particular staff members left, feeling angry, guilty, and inadequate. Still, problems remained. In fact, the staff turnover seemed to create more problems than it solved: cliques formed, both patients and staff members were made scapegoats, and unsubstantiated reports circulated about patients.

In order to understand the origin of the rumors, the unit's leaders made an extensive study of communications on the ward. A tape recorder was set up during nursing reports, and each communication was examined and compared with the events of the day as they had been observed and recorded. The study did shed some light on who started and spread the rumors and distortions about patients and staff members, but when the staff discussed these findings, their general attitude was that such events were natural and not amenable to correction.

Fifteen months after becoming director of the unit, the senior author left his position for one in research and training. Only after he was disengaged did he realize that he had been involved in the formation and development of a community. No longer the chief, he did not need to defend himself or, in the process, attack others. He was able then to return to the unit and observe, interview, and record the activities of the unit in the same way one would study any small society in an anthropological tradition. He was well aware that even as an observer he was not without bias. Yet, in his new role, physicians, staff, and patients became more trusting and therefore more willing to share confidences and feelings. From this perspective, a new view of the unit emerged.

Four or five years after it started, the unit came upon hard times. It had always had some difficulty in supporting itself because, though small, it required as many staff members as would a larger unit. Because staff relationships with private referring psychiatrists lacked clarity, staff members often were unfriendly toward and critical of some referring physicians. For example, when members of the nursing staff disapproved of the treatment plan of a senior psychiatrist, they often told him so in forceful terms; frequently, they actually subverted his plans. This happened most often to those physicians who treated patients with electroconvulsive or pharmacologic rather than psychotherapeutic means, since generally speaking they had lower status and found less favor with the staff. The physician with charm and the time to talk with the nurses, however, found he was welcome and his patients were well treated. Unfortunately for the life of the unit, it was the former kind of physician who most frequently hospitalized patients.

As private psychiatric units opened in other hospitals, and as these units made private physicians more welcome than the university unit did, psychiatrists began to refer their patients elsewhere. Consequently, the census of the unit dropped. During the last two years of its existence there were, on the average, far more staff members than patients on the ward at any one time. Finally, the unit was closed [1].

Nature abhors a vacuum. So do administrators. As it became apparent that the psychiatric unit would close, other departments moved to appropriate the space and resources. The winner was the Department of Physical Medicine and Rehabilitation, a division of the Department of Orthopedics. It seemed that a unit constructed for psychiatric patients would be well suited for patients with the chronic illnesses characteristic of the patient population of a rehabilitation unit. With almost no change in its physical structure except for installing telephones in the private bedrooms and placing railings and physical-therapy equipment in the dayroom, the new unit was opened in 1969.

Needless to say, one who had studied the psychiatric unit would look forward to making a comparative study of the rehabilitation unit. It would be the same size, have the same space, and, in some ways, have the same type of patients. Such a study in fact was made possible. Having been a consultant to the Department of Physical Medicine and Rehabilitation, the senior author of this book was invited to become the psychiatric consultant to the new unit.

The previous experience with the psychiatric unit enabled the new study to be approached far more methodically than the first had been. Observations of daily and special events were recorded from the inception. Contact with key staff was constantly maintained. Patients and staff were interviewed.

As time passed, we saw a repetition of the familiar struggles of staff and patients. The new unit began to experience census problems similar to those of the psychiatric unit. There were more staff members than patients, and the cost per patient day to the medical center became astronomical. Again, there was talk of closing the unit. Again, it proved to be more than talk, and the unit closed, four and one-half years after opening.

Colleagues who reviewed this manuscript have commented that an air of pessimism pervades it. If this is so, it probably derives from the fact that in the unit the ratio of patients with irreversible impairment to patients whose symptoms could be eliminated was very high. This issue is not dealt with in most therapeutic organizations, but instead is suppressed or dismissed as complaining, and it was not recognized as a major factor in determining morale in the subject unit.

Success produces rejoicing, self- and interperson- congratulation and camaraderie. The morale of a unit depends on the ratio of its successes to its failures. All-important is the definition of success. A hospice for the dying does not measure success by how many patients survive but rather by how comfortably they live as they approach death. A rehabilitation unit measures its success by how many patients it returns to function, to work, or to independent living.

The rehabilitation unit that is the subject of this report was a place to which only the most maimed and impaired were referred. The patients whose cases were simpler were treated as outpatients or referred to facilities in their own communities. Even the patients on this unit were sent to facilities in their communities or to their homes when they had improved, so that the full gratification that comes with dramatic positive change was denied the staff of the unit.

We disclaim pessimism about rehabilitation efforts, either with patients such as the ones described here or with rehabilitation subjects generally. But it is true that unless the special problems of rehabilitating a given population are recognized and understood, the staff will blame itself for not achieving what are in fact impossible goals.

1 The Idea of Therapeutic Environment

Therapeutic Environments

No society is without problems. Neither can any society tolerate having its problems stand before it, openly unalleviated. Societies, therefore, tend to seek solutions–restoration of function for the crippled, relief for the suffering, jail and reformation for the lawbreaker. The programs designed to solve human problems are demanded by the afflicted and the concerned, both of whom believe that where there is pain there must be a cure. Programs are supplied by the well-meaning and the self-seeking. Thus is created a group of professionals whose job is to propose and then implement solutions.

One of the solutions to human problems these professionals often propose is the specialized environment. Perhaps this is because environment is so frequently indicted as the source of success or failure in human affairs. We cite childhood environment as the cause of personality problems, or we credit it with the endowment of physical and mental strength. Poverty breeds antisocial behavior, affluence produces indolence, violence begets violence, compassion grows out of understanding–these are only a few of the environmental truisms to which we all refer.

The assumption underlying the specialized environment solution, then, is that just as certain environments are commonly acknowledged to be detrimental to health, so other environments will be therapeutic for certain types of individuals. If these individuals spend a given period of time in the specially designed environment, they will come out "better." Their improvement may be subjective in that they will feel better or believe they have progressed; and/or it may be objective in that those observing them will judge them to have improved. The area of improvement might be physical–increased strength, stamina, range of motion, or coordination–or it might be psychological and emotional–relief of anxiety, depression, fear, confusion, or a decrease in craving for substances such as drugs and alcohol. The improvement might also be social or moral–an increased willingness to conform to the laws of a community, or to fulfill the roles of a social group, or to adhere to religious principles and practices.

We find much experimentation in the pursuit of these optimally therapeutic environments. Our society, in fact, has a great many institutions that have been designated as therapeutic environments of one sort or another, therapeutic in the sense that certain persons would be "bettered" merely by their presence in them. These include not only psychiatric and rehabilitation units but also prisons, foster homes, boarding schools, and military services, among others. Also under the rubric of therapeutic environments come pain clinics, "fat farms," and hospital-prisons designed to cure as well as to contain those who have engaged in illegal sexual behavior.

Some of these solutions are indeed effective. Some are merely a placebo. And some of the solutions not only are unbeneficial, they are actually toxic—they exacerbate the problem they propose to cure. Because the range of the impact is so great, evaluation of the effectiveness of a given therapy or therapeutic environment is all important. Among several ways of evaluating a therapy, one way is to count cures. Cancer physicians, for example, speak of five-year survival rates. The effectiveness of antibiotics is evaluated by measuring the subsidence of fevers, the absence of bacterial growth on culture plates, and the relief of symptoms. The value of tranquilizers and antipsychotic agents is measured on similar scales.

However, as is well documented in volumes written on the problems of evaluating educational and therapeutic programs, evaluation on the basis of cures brings its own difficulties. There are many obstacles to effective measurement. One is methodological. For instance, we can measure an increase in reading skills, or arithmetical skills, or physical skills, but we cannot always demonstrate that their increase or decline came as the result of the interventions or the environment we designed. It is even more difficult to determine the history of more qualitative or ephemeral changes in attitude, motivation, mental health, and the like. The problems involved in accurately measuring progress are particularly relevant to rehabilitation programs where change is slow and painful and where success can mean growth but never cure.

Another obstacle to evaluating the impact of therapeutic environments can be found in the psychological and social predispositions of those concerned. Both those who supply and those who demand have difficulty in reasonable evaluation because they have an investment in believing a certain course of action to be effective. The supplier maintains his belief in his product's effectiveness both because in many cases he is part of the product he is selling (that is, the therapist) and because he profits from the sale. If he does not believe in what he sells, he must then see himself as a charlatan or confidence man, and most professionals have a variety of defenses against such a self-image.

The consumer, of course, also wants to believe in the effectiveness of a product, both because he wants a solution to a problem and because he does not want to feel that he has been cheated. In this way, the supplier (that is, the professional) and the consumer (that is, the afflicted or concerned) may end by collaborating in a process of mutual deception.

Problems in Rehabilitation

The rehabilitation unit is particularly susceptible to the problems of measurement described, and it is only reasonable to expect this to be true. Consider, after all, the particular situation of the rehabilitation patient. His is an extreme case of which we are all moderate examples. Any illness or disturbance of function, even the kind that results from dental extractions or, perhaps even more common, from learning that one must now and forevermore wear glasses, causes changes for the individual—changes in self-image, in self-esteem, in social relationships, and in feelings about the future. It often "shocks" the victim who, like all human beings, has tried to screen himself from the possibility that something bad could happen to him. It moves him from the ranks of the lucky to the ranks of the unlucky, to one of those persons marked for bad things—cancer, heart disease, permanent paralysis, or the like.

The ability to undo or reverse the bad effects of a natural event such as illness is important to man's psychological health. It is what gives him hope. Most frequently, of course, the reversal is possible, and with great relief the patient hears his orthopedist say that the leg, though fractured, will heal fully with no residual dysfunction. There are times, however, when the human body, as a result either of internal disease or of external trauma, is irreversibly altered. This is the predicament of the rehabilitation patient. Rehabilitation means problems, difficulties, limits, the inability to reverse the evil of illness.

This irreversibility causes further changes in the patient. Unlike those patients capable of recovery, rehabilitation patients often feel they have been banished. They feel they will never again have the same kinds of social relationships they once had; they will never again function in their former roles. They feel stigmatized and outcast. Thus, from the outset, their rehabilitation requires a major readaptation. They will have to form new self-concepts, social networks, and interpersonal relationships [2].

The process of rehabilitation, then, is highly complex, involving rehabilitation of the spirit as well as of the mind and body [3]. In practice, it means restoring function and structure, either naturally or artificially, through a training process in which the patient slowly learns new ways of performing basic functions. For example, a muscle that has not been used and that has become weak and small or limited in range of motion is both passively and actively mobilized until it reaches its new maximum level of function. An amputee is given a prosthetic device and taught to use it, being supported while he goes through the pain of adapting to it.

Rehabilitation of the spirit involves helping those who are paralyzed and profoundly depressed to overcome their emotional and physical sense of loss [4, 5, 6]. Through medications and psychotherapy the attempt is made to restore a natural outlook to the person who feels disfigured and therefore stigmatized by the community. This human being must be helped to believe once again that he has a place in his society, that he will be accepted by his community because he has a role to play.

Since the debilitating illness or trauma cannot be "cured," since the patient cannot literally be made whole again, the goals of rehabilitation medicine differ from those of other treatments. In psychiatry, for instance, we often witness the relief of symptoms. The psychological disturbance that caused the patient to be hospitalized disappears, and the patient is discharged. A success can be scored. In rehabilitation medicine, however, while symptoms subside during the primary phases, the basic work is to maximize function, to rehabilitate.

Because rehabilitation deals with function and not with symptoms [7, 8] and because each human being functions in a social and psychological as well as physical setting, the person-environment fit [9, 10, 11] is crucial. While the rehabilitation specialist can make predictions about the outcome of the physical rehabilitation effort, he has relatively little control over the environment. He can design a job for an injured person; he can prepare that person for the job; but he cannot create the job itself. Measuring the success of a rehabilitation unit, therefore, becomes far more difficult than evaluating the success of medical, surgical, or even psychiatric programs.

A rehabilitation program must work with practical definitions of success. In most cases, for instance, the rehabilitation program would not be expected to produce results that exceed the patient's premorbid level of performance. Previous experience also helps to determine what can be expected as an optimal outcome of treatment; for, while one sometimes meets with an outstanding rehabilitation patient who exceeds expectations, one never sees a miracle. A highly motivated patient or one who is very intelligent or financially well supported can, in an ideal environment, reach a higher level of performance than is normally expected. But from a practical viewpoint, most experts, after evaluating a rehabilitation patient, will concur on the maximum level of function that can be attained. Comparing the patient's performance following treatment with his premorbid performance, then, is one way of measuring the effectiveness of a rehabilitation unit. It focuses on the individual patient and the degree to which he approaches his own maximum level of functioning.

A second way of evaluating the effectiveness of a rehabilitation therapy is by comparing actual outcome with models of optimal and adverse outcome. For, as stated before, in rehabilitation there are no "cures," there are only positive and negative results. The following two hypothetical examples are extreme cases of optimal and adverse outcome. A thirty-one-year-old woman banged her wrist against a desk and suffered consequent swelling, pain, and guarding. There was no evidence of fracture or any significant damage. She was treated with pain medications, and as the pain diminished she was given physical therapy. After three weeks she was asymptomatic and had complete motion in her wrist. This is a model of optimal outcome. Contrast the experience of a twenty-eight-year-old woman who struck her wrist as she slipped on a ladder. There was some swelling, pain, and guarding. She was given pain medication and physical therapy, but her wrist became more painful and soon she could no longer move her hand and arm. A variety of specialists was unable to provide a diagnosis. Finally, neurosurgeons attempted to block the sympathetic nervous system to relieve the supposed cause of the dysfunction. Three years later, this woman's right hand was dysfunctional, atrophy had occurred, and eye and voice symptoms related to the sympathetic block appeared. This would certainly be a model of an adverse outcome.

Another way to measure the success of a therapeutic unit is to compare it to an alternative method of treatment. For example, the family could replace the hospital as a therapeutic setting. The following is an ideal instance of a family's rehabilitation effort. A twenty-eight-year-old accountant and auditor for a government agency was involved in an automobile accident, suffering multiple traumas to his body and brain. Comatose for a long period of time, he finally regained consciousness and recovered enough to be sent to a convalescent hospital. A short while after he had entered the hospital, the patient's parents became unhappy with his lack of progress and with the attitudes of the staff. They decided to bring him home. Through the workers' compensation agency, they hired an aide who would be responsible for continuing the patient's medical treatment, and the young man's father consulted a physiatrist, who offered some general guidelines for recovery. (The physiatrist in this case and in other rehabilitation cases usually integrates the medical care of the patient into a rehabilitative effort to restore function.) The physiatrist indicated how much could be done at home and what help could be given through the local community hospital. He suggested speech and occupational therapy that included restoration of self-care functions. The speech therapist suggested that someone read to the young man so he could start processing words and practice comprehending them. In addition, daily passive and active exercises were recommended. Based on the prescriptions of the experts, the man's parents established a full-time routine to achieve their goal of restoring their son to full function. The project became a challenge for the recently retired father and for the mother who, before the accident, had wondered what her future role would be. They became innovative and improved on the suggestions of the physiatrist and his staff. They invented special devices designed to develop self-care functions and worked with their son until he was able to perform them.

When we examined the patient approximately two years after the accident, he had indeed regained several functions: he was able to care for himself, to drive a car, and was sufficiently verbal so that it was possible to conduct a psychosocial evaluation of him with no difficulty. Some of the residual effects of the brain damage were evident, but in the opinion of the psychiatrist and all physicians involved, the results were remarkable. They were a far cry from the progress the patient had made while hospitalized and extended beyond the expectations of the medical specialists. This tremendous progress was made possible by the parents' devotion to and involvement with their son, and the personal meaning they themselves found in meeting the challenge.

This family approach to rehabilitation can be compared to programs in specially created social institutions such as hospital rehabilitation units, though when juxtaposed to the family just described, the comparison is not too favorable. The major distinction between family and institutional care is that the family establishes its rehabilitation program for one purpose only—to rehabilitate an individual who is very important to them. On the other hand, the hospital rehabilitation unit (in teaching hospitals particularly) is established to meet a spectrum of needs, including those of institutions, community, teachers, patients, and staff. In this sense, the rehabilitation of patients is not the exclusive objective of rehabilitation units. In fact, the general goal of a hospital rehabilitation unit often is to provide a place where the medical community or the community at large can send particular disabled persons for definitive evaluation, treatment, housing, planning, and disposition. Because of this, it is difficult to design an institution that provides an optimal social and psychological environment and virtually impossible to design one that provides the kind of love, care, interest, and direct participation that is found in the family.

It must be recognized, of course, that such a family as we have described is the exception, not the rule, and that the family also has a potential for destructive action. Some family members resent the great financial and physical burden involved and do not adjust well to having a disabled person to care for. Because their normal life-styles have been interrupted, they often make the injured person feel unwanted. Thus, we can again imagine two extreme examples of therapy and compare the relative success or failure of a hospital unit as it falls between the two.

The level of patient care, however, is not the only measurement applied when gauging the success of a therapeutic unit. Many other factors must be considered, as well. In the case of a teaching hospital, one would measure how well it accomplishes its job of teaching or research, as well as how effectively it provides quality patient care. Survival is another way of defining success. It is a cliché that all the world loves a winner and nobody likes a loser, and in relation to a rehabilitation unit, such a statement would be an exaggeration; but there is enough truth in the cliché to justify consideration. A unit's survival *may* coincide with its therapeutic success—or it may not. A unit could be very effective in treating patients; it could provide ideal teaching experience and high staff satisfaction; yet it could be nonlucrative or prohibitively expensive. Its survival could be determined by economic factors alone.

By the same token, many therapeutic environments survive and continue to operate with little consideration of how effectively they meet their goals. There is a common assumption that continued operation signifies success, and success means quality. Often, even the knowledge that the group is overstaffed or that certain individuals on the staff are incompetent cannot negate the operation=success=quality equation. It is not uncommon that mere survival is interpreted as success.

There are, of course, cases where a unit's survival does go hand in hand with its success or failure in meeting its objectives, in solving the problems it was designed to solve, in providing for the needs of those who work or study there, and in being economically solvent.

A Systems Approach

In evaluating and describing life on this rehabilitation unit, we have used a systems approach based on general systems theory. A systems approach views organizations as networks of interrelated elements [12, 13], interdependent at specific points. It identifies the units of an organization—the space, the people, the roles, the rules, the communication and leadership patterns—and it looks at how these interact. It examines the functions the organization must serve, and the values, practices, and techniques its members use to fulfill them; and it looks at all of these as they change and develop over time.

Underlying the systems approach is the assumption that in understanding an organization, personalities are far less important both for staff and patients than are roles and role functions. While this approach focuses on the expected and prescribed behavior of individuals, it also acknowledges the impact of diverse individual personalities and the multiple ways they will interact within the given roles. It acknowledges, for instance, that patients will differ greatly, that some may be placid and cooperative, others difficult and noncompliant. It understands that one staff person may show great initiative while another must constantly be given incentives to work. Yet while taking into account individual personality, the systems approach differs from a personality approach that looks at organizational behavior primarily in terms of the individual personalities of the participants. The systems approach looks at how these personalities interact with the system; it looks at them as elements in the system, always part of a wider field.

But, more importantly, the systems approach attempts to get away from simple cause-and-effect explanations, from exclusive focus on line- or step-reasoning. It recognizes that all organizations operate along numerous axes and that at any one time there are many interacting variables. To pick out any two and say they are causally related makes little sense. One must study all the relationships, and analyze these relationships as they evolve over time. No one person has that many eyes, so to speak, or that many ways of looking at a situation, so we try to study the whole in artificial ways. Like historians, we go back retrospectively, and after studying documents of what happened at a given time, we then try to reconstruct the situation based on information from various viewpoints and sources.

In evaluating a program like this rehabilitation unit, in trying to understand what happened, why it happened, and specifically why the unit failed, we will try to identify some of the numerous strands that went into both its life and its death.

There are several advantages to the systems approach. It forces the evaluator to be wary of simplistic common-sense explanations of what took place in one sphere of activity without going back to see what was happening within the whole system. For example, where it might seem that one person moved because he was pushed, a broader perspective could reveal that, in fact, there was another person on the other side pulling a string. This is the importance of the systems approach—one learns about the whole organization. A disadvantage of this approach is that as the number of variables is much greater, the conclusions are far less certain. The explanations, however, tend to be more valid and probably form a better basis for making predictions about the future.

There is another reason for using the systems approach—its emphasis is not on blame. This is not entirely true, of course, nor should one completely avoid finding fault. But in most instances, one cannot attribute to one piece of a system either the failure or the success of the whole organization. No single entity can explain the operation of the whole. The systems approach is a benign way of evaluating an organization, looking neither to condemn nor to give credit to any one individual. That it is benign does not alone make this approach worthwhile; that it is both benign and more valid recommends it as a tool for evaluation.

For the researcher, there is yet another reason to use the systems approach. It keeps him honest, in that he is forced to consider all the elements of the system—or at least as many as he can take in. When holding to a general systems philosophy, the researcher knows that when he answers to his critics (as all researchers must), they will be asking him, "Yes, but what about these other aspects of the organization? What was the impact of aspect Y or aspect Z, and how did it interact with ingredient A or B?" This helps the researcher design research that takes a larger number of parts into account, for he knows that unless he does, what he says may be valid but not necessarily relevant to an understanding of an organization. A researcher or evaluator can use a simple causal system to explain. He can say that A caused B, and it caused it every time; that inevitably when someone turned the key in the door, the door opened. But then one must ask, "So what? What does one learn from that?" Even though it may be a valid, predictable, reliable observation, it tells us nothing about how the whole building operated. The systems theory, then, encourages the researcher to take into account a broader range of observations in order to make both valid and relevant statements about an organization.

Finally, the systems approach permits the study of goals and objectives as they are related to the techniques or means available for achieving them. Most organizations, therapeutic units in this case, tend to describe themselves by their goals rather than by their achievements. In order to analyze what goes right or wrong, however, one must examine the means or components of a system. One can ask, for example, "Given these nurses, physicians, aides, what can be done to best rehabilitate the patients?"

The Design and Aims of the Study

These were some of the reasons why we have used, and are proposing further use, of the systems approach for the evaluation of organizations and, as we will later argue, for the planning of them, as well. In applying the systems approach to this study, it was clear to us that the failure of the unit, that is, its termination, could not be attributed to any individual action, but was a result of the nature of the system in which these individuals worked. Other personalities working in this setting would have faced the same problems, we felt, because the organizational system itself did not allow for effective functioning. As it is the environmental context that prohibits or permits certain types of behavior, we feel that if those persons on the unit had had a different set of directives they would have behaved differently, and perhaps the fate of the unit also would have been different.

Rather than offering a simple postmortem cause-and-effect explanation for the termination of the unit, one that attributes the result to the actions of an individual or of a particular event, this study seeks to understand the relationships among the different elements of the system. We will review and describe how the unit was planned, created, maintained, and phased out. We will show how the different parts of the picture interacted and how each part contributed to the whole. We will outline the inherent strains of the system that the individual personalities tried to cope with, and will show that the system did not have effective means for managing and bringing itself back in line when it ceased to function as planned. Without glorifying some or damning others, as would a personality-oriented approach [14], we will try to explain why an event happened or failed to happen by understanding the relationships within the structure of the whole system. We do this, of course, with the hope that by analyzing what failed, we may better understand how to design a rehabilitation unit or therapeutic environment that will not be plagued with the same problems.

Accepting the goals of rehabilitation—the physical and spiritual reintegration of the disabled individual within the community—as the core patient responsibilities of a rehabilitation unit, we then face the basic question of how. How do we design a unit that fulfills these functions maximally? How can we design a unit that at the same time cares for patients, trains staff to care for them, provides a basis for research, and offers opportunities for the growth and development of those working in the unit?

The unit examined here was part of a larger institution, a university teaching hospital. Because the investigators served as the psychiatric liaison service to this unit throughout its existence and were associated with the unit that preceded it, we were in an ideal position to conduct research. Through interviews and observations, we were able to know each patient and staff member. We were able to record how the unit was set up and to observe the problems that arose in administration, finance, staff organization, morale, and care of the patients.

Primarily using anthropological techniques, we studied the unit by taking the role of participant observers. The actual participants were more familiar with the specifics of the interactions on the unit, but they often had difficulty describing and evaluating it objectively. Paradoxically, the person with a greater understanding of the situation is also the one less knowledgeable about its particulars. The participant in a given situation is in a special position: he knows a great deal more about the situation and its history than the observer, but his objectivity is often clouded by his empathy and personal interest in it. He feels strongly about the other participants and is sensitive to whatever pain they might be experiencing. He may be angry at some and consider them "bad" people. Furthermore, the participant is sensitive to his own feelings. He may be hurt or angry or happy at what is taking place; he may believe that justice is triumphing or that evil has carried the day. And he reacts accordingly.

As participant observers, then, we tried to perceive the unit both through the perspectives of the various participants and through our own participation in the unit's activities, always stepping back to observe and analyze what we heard, saw, and experienced. In this book we have attempted to preserve these two perspectives. We have tried both to convey the perspective of the individual actors/participants by allowing them to speak for themselves about how they perceived the unit, and to step beyond the individual personalities of the situation and analyze the unit as a system composed of roles, rules, values, and communication and leadership patterns.

Also true to the anthropological tradition and in keeping with the systems approach, we looked at the unit both as a self-sufficient isolated whole composed of interrelated parts and as a unit that belonged to a larger whole of which it, too, was an integral part. Thus, on one level, we looked at the unit as if it were a small and definable island, even though its boundaries were highly permeable, with patients, staff, consultants, and visitors coming and going all the time. On another, we looked at it as a part of its larger setting, the hospital system, the community, and the society at large.

Because the unit was small, we were able to do a complete study. Unlike many medical anthropological studies of complex units or organizations, the study included interviews with everyone connected with the unit: the hospital administrator, members of the nursing administration, patients, and staff. In fact, over the four-year period, we interviewed most of them several times. Each person, obviously, had his own viewpoint about his specific role, and frequently these idiosyncratic responses were validated by others. More importantly, we were able to cross-validate the reports we received and thus never had to rely entirely on the testimony of a single informant.

We were not dependent upon the interviews alone. We also examined all available written materials: records of admission and discharge, notes of the nurses and physicians, documents on the goals and objectives of the unit, and descriptions of its operations, jobs, rules, and regulations.

Finally, we participated in, observed, and recorded all the types of behavior that took place on the ward. We recorded the formal behavior of the participants as they met together in conference or in treating a patient. We noted their informal behavior as they sat around the nursing station, the kitchen, or the dining area, and we observed forms of clan behavior at their parties, welcomings, departures, or holiday celebrations. We were privy to the attitudes and reactions of all the staff members and to those outside of the unit who interacted with them. And we did this throughout the entire life of the unit.

Agenda

This, then, is the theoretical and methodological background of this book. The planning and setting up of the rehabilitation unit, life on the unit, patient and staff roles and the values acted out through them, patient-staff interaction and the conflicts encountered, and some of the problems the unit faced as a system will be described. The "phasing out" stage of the unit from the perspective of both observers and participants will be presented, and the unit evaluated as to its therapeutic success.

We will simultaneously present what actually happened and how what happened contributed to the unit's success or failure, both in helping the individual patient and in fostering the unit's survival as an organization. By applying the systems approach postmortem, we hope to focus on those forces in the unit that foreshadowed its demise, and then to draw conclusions from these mistakes to guide in the planning and operation of other rehabilitation units. We will dissect all elements of the system: staff, patients, group interaction, and external and internal values that affected the implementation of the unit's goals. Each element, when taken as part of the whole, can provide us with a different perspective on how the unit operated and why it failed.

Recommendations will be offered on how to organize and operate a medical organization. A trouble-shooting system for identifying problems as they erupt will be described, and suggestions made for solving these problems. Needless to say, however, there are many "ifs" that must be inserted into any set of directives for planning and operating a medical unit.

This book proselytizes for a systems approach to medical organizations and emphasizes the importance of medical anthropologists helping medical administrators, hospital administrators, and physicians in dealing with the complex problems of treating patients in the hospital setting.

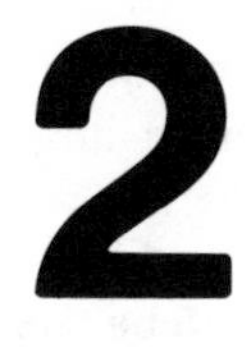

Planning and Setting Up the Unit

Need and Demand

A basic consideration in any planning situation is the demand for the projected services. Who is going to use them? Would they be used if given away free? Some things would not, jails, for instance. Some educational programs that are free, good, and ostensibly helpful to the public are underutilized or not utilized at all. Would the services be used if they were not free? The moment expense is added, the potential for utilization is reduced by the qualification of ability to pay.

One must clearly distinguish between need and demand. We may feel, for example, that people need education, or that they need psychotherapy. But, as we often discover to our discomfiture, what *we* feel people need may not coincide with what *they* feel they need. Demand, on the other hand, relates to the actual request for services and the actual use of services by those who can afford them.

Need and demand can be determined in a number of ways. Some large enterprises use market sampling to try to avoid misjudging demand and offering products or services no one will buy. Soap companies, for instance, try out their products ahead of time. They put new brands on the shelf, see how many are purchased, measure the consumer reaction, and in this way determine the demand.

Another way to determine demand, one more suitable to the purpose of implementing a rehabilitation unit, uses an experiential approach. Someone working in the field, in a hospital setting, perhaps, sees that people need a certain service, that there are many instances in which it would be used were it available. On the basis of this, the person says, "Let's create this service and I predict people will use it, because I've already seen so many who needed it." This experiential approach to demand was, in fact, instrumental in the creation of the rehabilitation unit.

Another way of determining need and demand involves an aesthetic approach analogous, for example, to saying of a picture: "What this picture needs to be complete is a cloud in that corner, or a flower, or some additional piece of green. It would fit. It's necessary." Similarly, in evaluating the services provided by an institution, planners say, "In order to provide complete services one should have this additional unit. The hospital needs it. And it would fit." This also was one of the justifications used for forming the rehabilitation unit.

What, then, were some of the needs the planners wanted this unit to meet? First, there were the needs of patients who remained hospitalized after the acute phase of their illness, patients whose further care was primarily reconstitutive rather than medical. For example, an amputee would be fitted with a new prosthetic device and taught how to use it, or he would be taught new skills and how to reeducate his muscles.

In general, these patients were kept in the hospital because it was inconvenient for the professionals caring for them to go to their homes. Although there seems to be a pervasive fantasy that a house call by a health professional is the best and most desirable way to treat a patient, home visiting is, by and large, a very expensive proposition, utilizing costly professional time. On a large scale it is far more practical to bring the nonproductive sick person to the productive health professional than vice versa.

So, although these patients could not be sent out of the hospital without further treatment, it was not feasible to treat them at their homes. They had either to be brought daily to the hospital or somewhere else for professional treatment, or receive no treatment at all. Most people who lived in the vicinity of the hospital or close to the medical center could manage to travel back and forth on this daily basis by the various means available—vans that take wheelchairs, ambulances, or other vehicles specially adapted for disabled or rehabilitation patients. But for those patients (and there were many) who lived some distance from the center, daily transport could become much too expensive and time-consuming. It was partly this need for a place where certain patients could be kept for further care more conveniently and economically than they could be kept on the acute hospital services that the planners considered when they said, "We need a rehabilitation unit."

Also, extended hospitalization for rehabilitation patients created problems for the hospital. Although this is no longer the case nationally, the beds in many hospitals, and in this one especially, were then at a premium (as the hospital is subsidized, the factors of demand change somewhat). The patient using an orthopedic or neurosurgical bed while being rehabilitated prevented another orthopedic or neurosurgical patient from entering. This, too, was part of the pressure for a rehabilitation unit.

Thirdly, there were people in the community who were not receiving care because such a unit was not available. The various convalescent hospitals that existed in the community were not convalescent hospitals in the strictest sense of the term, because they did not really provide extended-care facilities. Originally, these hospitals had been created for patients who, because of their physical and/or mental state, were unable to function at home on their own. While they did need some additional care, it was not the kind offered by a general hospital. These "convalescent" hospitals had in fact become more or less "storage" facilities for old people. Admitting a patient into one of them might be more destructive than therapeutic, and they were not considered good rehabilitation environments. This situation imposed further pressure for the creation of a rehabilitation unit.

Finally, it was felt that a rehabilitation unit would play an important role in the training of the various health-care professionals on the medical-university campus: nurses, pharmacists, physical therapists, medical students, and others. On an aesthetic basis, the notion existed that "people should have this kind of training," although it was not certain what the actual demand would be for the special training if it were offered.

Objectives

There were certain core functions the proposed unit would have to serve in order to survive, and certain components were required to perform these functions.

The functions or objectives of the unit were: (1) to provide a place where the physically handicapped and disabled could be evaluated and treated; (2) to accept enough physically handicapped and disabled persons for evaluation and treatment so the unit would not be seen as overselective or as not meeting the needs of the community it was created to serve; (3) to satisfy the referring physicians that the unit was fulfilling its role; (4) to satisfy the supporting agencies, including, in some instances, the families of patients, that the unit was performing as desired; (5) to satisfy hospital agencies, such as utilization review boards, that the services provided were ones that could be delivered only in that place at that cost; (6) to manage a patient-rehabilitation unit separation in as mutually satisfying a way as possible; that is, patients could not just be released when they were finished with hospital treatment–someone had to find a suitable place that would be acceptable to the patient, the community at large, the families, the referring physicians, and other interested parties; (7) to occupy the patients' time in a reasonably meaningful way while they were on the unit; (8) to be humane to the patients; and, finally, (9) to practice in accordance with community standards, to avail themselves of all the resources the medical center and the community had to offer.

In order to meet these requirements the proposed unit needed: (1) a place; (2) a staff with the proper distribution of professionals readily available for consultation; (3) referrals (that is, patients sent by someone); (4) intrastaff communication and cooperation; (5) the goodwill of those outside the unit; and (6) a positive community image of the unit's function, that is, a general approval of the operation, even by those who knew little of what specifically was being done.

Generally speaking, those who designed the unit hoped it would provide a therapeutic environment, not only in the narrow physical sense, but in the broader psychological and social sense as well. However, there was no specific planning for assuring that the unit would be socially and psychologically therapeutic; the general notion was never verbalized, nor was there ever any analysis, any detailing, or any consideration of how, in fact, the unit would be socially and psychologically therapeutic. It was thought that some analysis of a patient's social situation would be done by a social worker. It was thought that psychiatric consultation might be utilized to take care of any psychological problems. But basically there was only a hope and a faith that with well-trained people who were helpful, good, and kind, there would be a beneficial social and psychological effect on the patients in the unit.

Planning

The layman—by which we mean the person who is not professionally or technically involved in an enterprise—frequently, if not always, assumes that the designers have given more thought, analysis, and discussion to planning and design than they actually have done. In the formation of this particular unit, there was far less thinking-through or systems-planning than might have been expected.

There were a number of givens, one of which was space, and there were some alternatives as to how that space might be arranged. One room could be made into a treatment room, another could be used for a dining room, but there were limits to the changes possible. Beyond the givens, however, there were many contingencies that the planners did not visualize, many problems they did not know were going to occur. They planned structurally rather than functionally, thinking of numbers and kinds of patients and staff members, rather than of how these would interact. In effect, they said, "In this rehabilitation unit, we will need a physiatrist, someone who is a specialist in physical medicine and rehabilitation. We're certainly going to need nurses, because we're going to have medically ill patients. We're going to need one or more physical therapists because we're going to need someone who can do physical therapy. We're going to need an occupational therapist because these are people who specialize in teaching people to do tasks, and we want to integrate that into our organization."

All of this thinking was in fixed terms that did not take into consideration how these people were going to interact with each other, how they were going to grow and to treat each other, or how well suited they were for life on the unit. The plans were all based on structure rather than dynamic function. Because the thinking was wholly structural, it left out one important ingredient that could not be specifically predicted at the design stage—namely, personality.

There are several possible reasons why there was so little thinking-through in the planning and setting up of this unit. First, it is quite possible that because the planners were given a set space rather than being allowed to design one, they were inhibited from working through the details of other aspects of the design, perhaps feeling it was not necessary. It is possible, for example, that had they been given a sum of money and told, "We're going to allocate X millions of dollars for you to design and build a rehabilitation unit," they would have looked far more closely at every aspect of the architectural design. And in analyzing carefully the architectural design, they would have been forced to think of the people who would be going into the structure. The planners would then have had to imagine where the patients and the staff were going to move, what their roles would be, how and where they would interact. This might have helped them to think in systems terms, to think through the design of the unit as an integrated whole and to imagine how it would function. But this was not the case. Instead, the planners took over a finished structure; their space was a given and the opportunities for change were few.

A second difficulty arose because there was no precedent for the unit, nor were there people available with experience working in a twenty-four-hour-a-day residential rehabilitation environment. Although the campus had operated an outpatient rehabilitation clinic utilizing rehabilitation specialists, there never had been an inpatient rehabilitation unit. Furthermore, there were no other such units in the community. In starting a new unit like this one, people usually go out and learn from or copy other, established, organizations. As no model of a rehabilitation unit existed in this community, the planners did not have access to the valuable information that comes from experience.

The rehabilitation unit was to be unusually small. Most formal rehabilitation units in the country, such as the Veterans Administration units, are much larger than the nine-bed unit with which we are concerned. Generally, they serve twenty, thirty, or forty patients. In this respect, also, there were no relevant models for the design. Perhaps the planners did not actually ask, "Is there a model we can use?" but the lack of such a model must be considered as part of the problem.

Two other general problems—problems of human nature—often hamper good planning because they interfere with the use of others' experience. First of all, it may not be enough to tell someone that a kind of problem exists or might exist. He may be unable to make use of this information unless he has experienced the problem himself and has conceptualized and studied the experience. Second, it may be difficult for planners to foresee the kinds of difficulties that may occur, because they have never before encountered them. Both of these problems were present in the planning of the rehabilitation unit—the difficulties that arose were not foreseen and the planners, who had not been involved with the previous psychiatric unit, were unable to imagine that the experience of that unit might be applicable to the new unit.

The Unit in the Hospital Setting

When we discuss environmental impact, it is all too easy to consider the relationship of a unit to the neighborhood in which it is placed rather than to the immediate environment in which it functions. The success or failure of a given medical treatment project may, in fact, be more dependent on its micro-environment, on its relations to other existing units and persons in the hospital, than it is on the physical environment, the neighborhood that surrounds it.

The establishment of a new patient care unit within a general hospital may add or take away resources from other units, eliciting support or antagonism from those tangentially involved, or it may cause a disturbing or healthy traffic flow within the hospital. Contrarily, the hospital may add or take away resources from the new unit, either helping it to flourish or making survival difficult. In any case, it sets the ground rules upon which the unit must function.

This rehabilitation unit was intimately connected with its micro-environment, first and most importantly through its attachment to the hospital administration. It was by no means an autonomous unit. The chancellor, the dean, the hospital administrator, the chairman of the Department of Orthopedics, and the director of nursing all participated in the birth, life, and death of this unit.

In a university hospital, it is the chancellor and the dean who decide whether or not a new unit is necessary, and it was they who made the initial decision that the rehabilitation unit should exist. Involved in the implementation of this decision were the hospital administrator, the chairman of the Department of Orthopedics, and the man who was selected to be the ward director. The hospital administrator was primarily responsible for the practical problems of the unit, for all channels of money, personnel, and supplies that went in and out of it. The dean was responsible for the students and teachers involved. The chairman of the Department of Orthopedics had the most immediate authority over the ward director, and the subordinates of both the hospital administrator and the chairman worked out the practical details and problems of starting and running the ward. The director of nursing approved the assignment of nurses to the unit.

The rehabilitation unit was linked with its micro-environment in a second way, in that each staff person on the unit was also identified and sometimes primarily identified with a service outside of the unit. A rehabilitation ward in a university hospital is not like a private rehabilitation center. Each nurse is ultimately under the supervision of the director of nursing as well as immediately answerable to the head nurse of the unit. Each physician belongs to a particular department, and each physical therapist has a chief outside the ward. No one belongs solely to the rehabilitation unit. Inevitably, problems will arise because of this fragmentation of authority. The attitudes or prejudices of the unseen bosses may be reflected by their employees who work on the unit; in fact, it would be difficult to imagine an employee not being influenced in some way by the attitudes of those under whom he works. But as these influences are seldom overt, they cannot be readily identified or confronted. Often one member of the staff will feel constraints about cooperating with a program because he does not have the approval of his outside chief. Further, he does not wish to say that he is dependent on that approval, an action that might direct criticism toward himself or the unseen chief. As a result, he may appear uncertain and indecisive, when in fact he is not clear about his orders. Ideally, of course, both unit and hospital administration will be working toward the same goals in the same way, and then no division of loyalty will occur. But ideal is seldom real, and conflict of interest can become a major obstacle to the operation of a unit that is not autonomous.

A third way in which the unit was affiliated with the larger hospital setting was in the requirement that it reflect the hospital's policies regarding staff rights, staff behavior, and the general prevailing culture of medicine. The unit could not simply institute its own set of rules and regulations, and this became particularly important in connection with staff rights and staff behavior. The autocratic system in which hiring and firing was the right of the administration, with the staff member having little control over his own destiny, had been replaced by a system in which grievance procedures protected the staff member from a whimsical authority. Committees composed of the staff member's peers and sometimes his supervisors and subordinates gave the final verdict on the discharge of a worker, and an employee could no longer be fired without good cause. The drawback to this system was that even when the administration could demonstrate sufficient cause, a sympathetic committee could reverse its recommendation. As a result, and as we will later see was the case on this unit, administrators often had to learn to work with staff whom they did not respect or trust, but who were not flagrantly incompetent or abusive of patients.

Situated within the university hospital, the unit seemed to be a part of the hospital community, part of a group with a shared identity, shared values, and shared work experience. However, the unit had characteristics that made entry into the hospital community difficult, because in many ways, rehabilitation units, like psychiatric units, differ from other hospital units. Staff on both of these wards operate in a rhythm different from that of medical surgical units. With the tendency toward a constant population, the pace of the staff seems leisurely compared with the more pressured tempo of the acute care units. Also, rehabilitation staffs employ many specialists—physical therapists, nurses, specialty and vocational therapists, and psychotherapists—and so tend not to be so cohesive a group as staff on other units might be. Finally, rehabilitation units are generally small and self-contained, geared to be more autonomous than other units.

Physical Design

It is impossible to ignore the systemic impact of milieu (the structural and design aspects of the unit) on treatment [15]. The physical environment of this ward, particularly the arrangement of space, was indeed a vital part of the unit's total therapeutic environment.

The ward was fairly spacious, though not intentionally so. Its former usage as a psychiatric unit resulted in its being equipped with room for a shuffleboard, piano, and other play and therapy equipment. It was also the only ward with its own kitchen, hairdressing, and laundry facilities, all suited for developing a total therapeutic community. A small dining room provided a common eating area for the patients as well as a visiting area for friends and relatives, and a social room was available for watching television and doing mat exercises (see figure 2–1). Most physical-therapy sessions, however, also took place in the social room even though there was an outpatient rehabilitation center downstairs in the hospital basement, and this created potential conflicts.

The fact that the rehabilitation ward was virtually isolated from other wards in a westerly wing encouraged the development of a separate culture. Double doors led to the entrance of the unit, cutting it off from another private ward nearby. The ward contained nine private rooms, each with bed, nightstand, chair, wardrobe, and telephone. While these bedrooms gave the patients privacy, they also isolated the patients from one another. Privacy is considered desirable [16], especially for ambulatory patients, but for patients who are physically disabled and often bedridden, the private room can become a prison cell. The two-bed room or the four-bed room, on the other hand, provides relief from isolation, for patients can talk to each other, but it may present the opposite problem of too little privacy.

In many ways this ward was unique. People did not wander through it—there was no through passageway. When the doors were closed, the ward became a special, private sector enjoyed by both patients and staff. There was no rush, no obvious confusion, and no visible upset. People could not enter without being conspicuous, yet the ward was conveniently situated only five feet from the hospital's major elevator. The fact that there was no through passageway did mean, however, that the patients were not likely to mix with patients or staff from other units. Thus, while privacy was retained, the opportunities for outside company and exchange were few.

The unit still bore the physical marks of its former usage as a psychiatric unit. The windows were supposedly suicide proof (although they were not in fact so), and this contributed to the sense of the ward's physical isolation. Also, the nursing station had been constructed like the old state hospital psychiatric stations, with surrounding glass so that the patients outside could be observed, while the staff inside were protected from intrusion and could not be heard by those outside. This allowed staff on the unit, particularly on the night shift, to go inside the station and get away from the patients. The passage into the station was not wide enough to admit a wheelchair.

The main corridor of the ward was not really visible from the nursing station, and the corridor was a dead-end, further emphasizing the isolation of the ward from the rest of the hospital. Going out required going through another unit's corridor, going up or down an elevator, down another corridor, and then

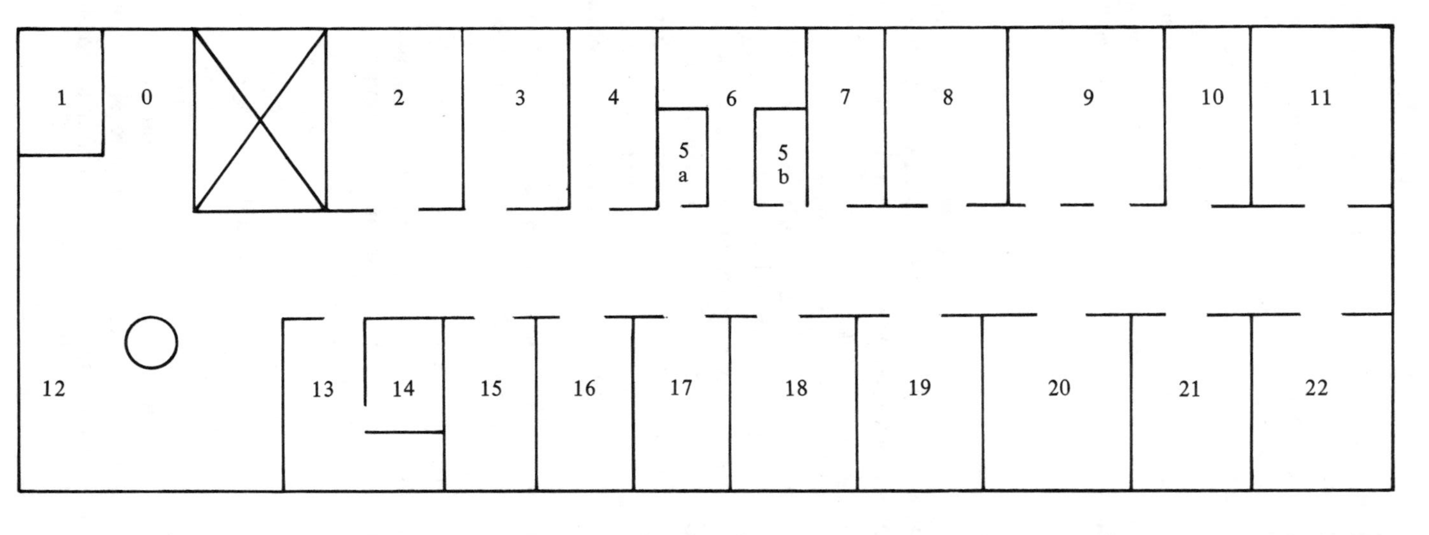

Source: From K.W. Payne, "The Culture of a Small Rehabilitation Ward." Unpublished paper. University of California, San Francisco, 1973.

0 Entrance and Exit to Ward 3–1, Rehabilitation
1 Staff Toilet
2 Kitchen
3 Utility Room
4 Small Linen Closet
5a–b Patients' Toilet
6 Patients' Shower (Left) and Bathtub (Right)
7 Cloak and Supply Room
8 Private Bedroom
9 Dining Room
10 Emergency Exit and Passage
11 Laundry Room
12 Day Room
13 Nursing Station
14 Head Nurse's Office
15–22 Private Bedrooms

Figure 2-1. Time Spent in Rehabilitation Unit (hours per week) by Role Designation

out a door. Once outside, there was no garden area or other place where a disabled person could safely move about.

The design features of the ward also set specific limits on the number and kinds of patients who could be treated there, thus limiting the community of the ward. There were no isolation rooms for patients with contagious illnesses. There were no air outlets for oxygen, making it very difficult to accommodate patients with lung or respiratory problems; and the absence of bathrooms and wash basins in the rooms meant that there were no facilities for discarding of wastes, eliminating as members of the unit any patients with communicable diseases.

The Rehabilitation Patient

Rehabilitation patients are defined by social standards. Persons who are dying are not considered rehabilitation patients, while persons who would get well even without rehabilitation efforts sometimes are. The criteria often depend on how much society is willing to invest to bring disabled persons back to maximum physical and psychological strength. Society sets a price on its rehabilitation goals, the price varying with the time and the person [17]. For instance, governments usually are willing to spend their money on veterans but not on those who become ill or who have been injured outside of war or industry. Industry, in turn, is required to spend money to rehabilitate workers who have been injured on the job [18], but that is where its responsibility ends. Families, on the other hand, would ask society to invest everything necessary to restore a family member's health.

Within the hospital setting, the rehabilitation unit received its patients from wards that could no longer help them. Patients with incurable skeletal, muscular, or neurological diseases and defects or irreparable spinal-cord injuries were the candidates for rehabilitation here. The recruitment process started with referral by a physician in another service or by an outside physician. The ward director would be called in as a consultant to advise on the case, and admission procedures would follow if the patient was deemed appropriate.

Inasmuch as this was a closed ward, admissions were selective and all patients were screened. A closed ward, by definition, is one that accepts only certain patients. Either because it is highly specialized in skills or techniques, or because it believes it cannot help some patients, or because it believes that certain patients would be disruptive to the staff and patients already on the unit, a closed ward ideally will study its prospective patient carefully before admitting him. Thus, a patient who is psychotic might be excluded from a rehabilitation unit, whereas a patient who is not psychotic might be excluded from a psychiatric unit.

When there were enough patients available, the ideal was invoked and preference was shown for younger and less disabled persons. When there was a shortage of patients, a condition that became more common than exceptional toward the end of the ward's life, the criteria for admissions became less selective. Initially, only those patients were chosen who showed promise for success and whose therapeutic needs fitted the particular facilities offered by the unit.

Several kinds of criteria were invoked in the selection process. These differed among the various professionals who worked on the ward, each having his own concept of the "ideal patient" for the unit that was based partly on his knowledge of the course of certain disabilities and partly on his own personality and work interests. The unlikelihood that any two, three, or four staff members would agree that the same patient qualified as ideal made consensus in selection difficult, and it was often the case that part of the staff were unhappy with the patient population selected.

This was particularly true of the nurses who, more than any other staff group, carried the greatest burden in caring for the patients. Most nursing-staff members preferred the patient whose illness was controllable and uncomplicated and whose course of illness was predictable. They seldom appreciated those patients who, in addition to their obvious orthopedic-related disabilities, had emotional problems, postoperative complications (hemorrhages, coronaries, and so forth), or special complications such as diabetes or other diseases. Caring for these complications would be mainly the nurses' responsibility. Since this particular rehabilitation unit was not equipped to care for certain medical problems such as respiratory illnesses or infectious illnesses, the nurses were vehemently opposed to the admission of patients suffering from any of those complications and, in one instance, the head nurse refused to accept a patient who had been approved by the patient's physician and the ward director.

From the nurses' perspective, the ideal patient generally could be described as one who makes staff members feel good by being cooperative and by not challenging them [19, 20]. The patient should seem to make progress, or if he makes no progress, at least he should not complain or blame the staff. In fact, they might feel that the "uncooperative" patient should simply be denied rehabilitation services.

The ward director, on the other hand, was obligated both to fill the beds and to fill them with patients who had teaching significance. He could not admit patients whose infirmities were too similar, but had to see that the patient population represented a spectrum of disabled cases.

The potential patient's motivation was a perhaps less apparent but very important criterion for selection, and it was one shared by all the staff [21]. The staff did not take much serious interest in anyone who came to the ward without the motivation to improve his condition. Often, a patient lacking motivation was admitted but not accepted as part of the ward community.

Patients were closely observed in an effort to determine what motivation existed and what the inhibitors to it might be [22]. For example, depression might block a patient's motivation or a patient might resist therapy because he had difficulty accepting any sort of organization or routine. The treatment, then, would have to take these inhibiting factors into consideration, since any successful therapy would require that the emotional difficulties be confronted.

A second criterion was that patients should be selected for whom there was hope, and that those who aroused too much feeling or empathy should be rejected. Dying patients, the ones obviously unlikely to survive their disabilities, understandably were not considered good rehabilitation candidates. Rehabilitation staffs like to see themselves as professional groups who produce change for the better. The humanitarian act of maximizing ability while a person is dying is not included in the staff member's image of his role.

Of the patients who were selected for treatment on the unit (664 in the four and one-half years of its existence), about 73 percent (481) were core or "regular" patients. As a group these were the truly disabled, the truly impaired, the truly traumatized. They were the ones who could not move out of bed by themselves, the ones who were truly dependent on others for every aspect of supply and for every aspect of function. They needed their food to be brought to them, and some needed to be fed. Some needed to be clothed, some needed to be bathed, and some could not attend to bladder or bowel functions, either because they were neurologically impaired or because they could not move to the bathroom. Almost all the rehabilitation patients had one or more of the following conditions: hemiplegia (a unilateral paralysis which, in most cases, had resulted from trauma or a cerebrovascular accident or stroke); amputation of one or both lower extremities, either above or below the knee; a spinal-cord injury resulting in measurable paralysis; multiple sclerosis; rheumatoid arthritis; or complicated fractures (table 2-1). As this particular ward was specifically oriented toward the treatment of patients from orthopedics and neurosurgery, it did not admit those who were blind, patients with upper extremity problems, drug addicts, or those with mental disturbances.

About 27 percent (180) of the total patient population were seen for Nevada Industrial Commission workups (NIC patients) and these could not be classified as rehabilitation patients. Important to the financial stability of the unit, these admissions were under the director's control and could be scheduled in advance when a vacancy or low-occupancy period was expected. NIC patients were not a strain on the staff since no special provisions had to be made for them, but the nurses found them undesirable because they required a great deal of paper work and no treatment. They were held suspect by some of the staff, who thought it possible that many of them had severe cases of contentionitis; that is, they were thought to be exaggerating their disabilities in order to collect the greatest possible compensation [23]. This, understandably, was forbidden on a ward where patients were truly disabled and were supposed to emphasize functional parts and health rather than disability and illness. Instances such as one female NIC patient's telling the head nurse, "I've got to get back to my bed and play crippled," reinforced the staff's mistrust. They felt these patients had an antitherapeutic influence on the ward. NIC patients did, however, prove to be good teaching patients, both for students and residents, as a contrast to the severely injured patients who formed the core group of the rehabilitation unit.

Over the years (table 2-2), the number of NIC patients admitted to the unit increased while the population of "regular" rehabilitation patients declined, and the emphasis on the rehabilitation ward shifted slowly away from regular rehabilitation (in 1969 about 88 percent of the patients were there for rehabilitation therapy and 10 percent for NIC and compensation workups) toward NIC patient care (in 1973 about 60 percent of the patients were admitted for rehabilitation and 40 percent for NIC and related workups). The average length of stay for the regular rehabilitation patient ranged from 24.2 days in 1969 to 12.7 days in 1973 (table 2-3). NIC patients averaged only 2.3 days because they were admitted just for evaluation, and only a short stay was necessary for the careful coordination of their workups. Age is considered a prime determining factor in rehabilitation [24], and rehabilitation teams are known to have strong, overt biases in favor of youth. However, as seen in table 2-4, the average age of the patients on this rehabilitation unit was 54.2 years. The youngest patient was fourteen, and the oldest was eighty-eight. The sex balance on the ward was fairly even (tables 2-3, 2-4, 2-5, 2-6).

Once eligibility for rehabilitation had been determined, the patient underwent a diagnostic and evaluative process. This process was intended to determine the severity of the patient's disability and the possibility or practicality of alternative programs [25]. Interviews and a series of tests were used to reveal the patient's "potential." Counseling interviews and individual program-planning then followed, and during this process the patient ostensibly was involved in determining his future hospitalization goals. It was during these interviews (as well as continuously thereafter) that the required motivation on the part of the patient was carefully determined.

Generally, the patient was enlisted only informally in the planning for his treatment and rehabilitation. Often he was so overwhelmed by what had happened to him that he could focus on only one aspect of his rehabilitation and tended to ignore the rest. Also, it was easier to talk about a patient when he was not there and, as a result, most planning was done in the patient's absence. Families sometimes were enlisted in the planning effort, and both the patient and his family were invited to the rounds at which the patient would be discussed [26]. However, very little time was assigned to the consideration of each patient in these rounds and the enlistment of the family was frequently no more than a token gesture.

Following the formation of the treatment schedule, the plan was implemented and then checked for unforeseen problems. From time to time the case

Table 2-1
Number of Patients with Specific Diseases and Illnesses
(In decreasing order of frequency on the ward)

	1969	*1970*	*1971*	*1972*	*1973*[a]	*1969-1973*
Back Pains and Back Trouble (Lower Back Pains and Cervical-Lumbar Pains	19	32	48	50	28	177
Amputation (Lateral)	17	11	7	8	5	48
Hemiparesis	6	6	16	15	5	48
Paraplegia	10	13	8	10	2	43
Rheumatoid Arthritis	7	7	14	7	3	38
Fractures (Complex)	6	1	11	7	3	28
CVA (Cerebral Vascular Accident, Stroke, Cerebral Thrombosis, and Aneurysms)	9	5	2	4	2	22
Paraparesis	8	3	5	3	3	22
Quadriplegia	3	5	7	5	1	21
Weakness (Generalized or Lateral)	3	3	3	6	2	17
Hemiplegia	5	4	3	4	1	17
Knee Injury or Problem	0	4	7	4	2	17
Neck Injury	1	4	3	6	3	17
Hip Problem	3	1	3	5	2	14
Amputation (Bilateral)	4	0	5	2	1	12
Quadriparesis	4	1	2	3	2	12
Head Injury	1	4	1	2	3	11
Total Hip Replacement	0	2	3	1	4	10
Laminectomy	2	3	2	2	0	9
Brain Tumor	2	1	1	2	3	9
Shoulder Injury or Problem	2	0	3	3	1	9
Spinal Cord Compression	5	0	1	1	0	7
Spinal Fusion	1	3	1	1	1	7
Arthritis	0	0	3	3	1	7
Multiple Sclerosis	5	0	2	0	0	7
Aphasia	1	0	2	1	2	6
Brain Stem Tumor or Injury	0	2	1	2	1	6
Spinal Injury (Unspecified)	0	1	3	0	1	5
Ankle Injury or Problem	0	0	2	3	0	5
Herniation of Nucleus Pulposus	1	1	1	2	0	5
Post Polio Disability	2	1	0	1	0	4
Craniotomy	0	2	1	1	0	4
Degenerative Disc Disease	0	0	2	2	0	4
AV (Arterial-Venous) Malformation	0	0	3	0	1	4
Hand Surgery or Problem	0	0	3	1	0	4
Neuropathy	3	1	0	0	0	4
Cardiac Arrest (Myocardial Infarction; Heart Attack)	3	0	0	0	0	3
Diabetes	1	1	1	0	0	3
Hemipelvectomy	0	0	2	1	0	3
Osteo-Arthritis	0	0	2	1	0	3
Comprehensive Workup (No Specific Complaint Given)	3	0	0	0	0	3
Parkinson's Disease	0	2	0	0	0	2

Table 2-1 Continued

	1969	*1970*	*1971*	*1972*	*1973*[a]	*1969-1973*
Polyneuritis	0	1	0	1	0	2
Ankylosing Spondylitis	0	1	1	0	0	2
Cerebral Contusion	2	0	0	0	0	2
Chest Injuries	0	0	1	0	1	2
Convulsive Disorders	1	0	0	1	0	2
Foot Operation	0	0	1	1	0	2
Arm Injury	0	1	1	0	0	2
Hematomas	0	1	1	0	0	2
Hodgkin's Disease	2	0	0	0	0	2
Mastectomy	0	1	0	1	0	2
Spinal Cord Tumor	0	0	2	0	0	2
Pelvic Injury	0	1	0	0	0	1
Pseudo Arthrosis	1	0	0	0	0	1
Pott's Disease (TB of Spine)	0	0	0	1	0	1
Pyelonephritis	1	0	0	0	0	1
Radiation Myelopathy	1	0	0	0	0	1
Scleroderma	0	0	1	0	0	1
Spondylosis	1	0	0	0	0	1
Stump Revision	1	0	0	0	0	1
Stump Problem	0	1	0	0	0	1
Brown-Sequard Syndrome	1	0	0	0	0	1
Burns	0	0	1	0	0	1
Electric Shock	0	0	0	1	0	1
Flexion Contracture	1	0	0	0	0	1
Airway Obstruction	0	1	0	0	0	1
Ambulation Disability	0	1	0	0	0	1
Knee Arthroplasty	1	0	0	0	0	1
Bleeding Ulcer	1	0	0	0	0	1
Mulcular Dystrophy	0	0	1	0	0	1
Neurogenic Bladder	1	0	0	0	0	1
Organic Brain Syndrome	0	1	0	0	0	1
Palsy	1	0	0	0	0	1
TEA (Thrombo-End-arterectomy)	1	0	0	0	0	1
Tendon Transplant	0	1	0	0	0	1
Torn Ligament	0	1	0	0	0	1
Arm Tendonitis	0	0	1	0	0	1
Spinal Cord Transection	1	0	0	0	0	1
Tumor of Head	0	1	0	0	0	1
Urinary Infection	1	0	0	0	0	1

This table was compiled by nursing staff.
[a]January–April only.

would be discussed at Grand Rounds, where staff met to go over the events of the week, and the success or failure of the patient's treatment would be reviewed.

While treatment was still being given, a discharge plan would also be evolving. The time of discharge usually was based on two elements: first, the expected and achieved level of maximum performance and, second, the patient's re-

Table 2–2
Categorical Differences in Patient Types Over Time

	1969	*1970*	*1971*	*1972*	*1973*[a]	*1969–1973*
Total Number of Patients (all types)	133 (100%)	125 (100%)	167 (100%)	169 (100%)	70 (100%)	664 (100%)
I. Number of Regular (non-NIC) Patients	177 (88%)	92 (74%)	114 (68%)	116 (69%)	42 (60%)	481 (73%)
II. Number of NIC Patients	13 (10%)	33 (26%)	53 (32%)	53 (31%)	28 (40%)	180 (27%)
III. Number of Patients with Undetermined Status	3 (2%)					

[a]January–April only.

sources—private, insurance, or public. In order to determine the resources, the social worker surveyed all potential sources of income. When the family was involved and the patient had reached his rehabilitation goal, the patient was discharged directly into the family setting. However, there sometimes were conflicts between a patient's readiness to leave and a community's or family's willingness to receive the patient. As a result, some patients needed room and

Table 2–3
Average Length of Stay on the Rehabiliation Ward, by Patient Type and Sex
(In days)

	1969	*1970*	*1971*	*1972*	*1973*[a]	*1969–1973*
Average Stay (All patients)	22.0	25.6	11.5	13.0	8.4	16.3
Male	23.3	21.2	12.2	14.1	8.0	16.3
Female	20.5	34.7	10.6	11.6	8.8	16.3
I. Average Stay for a Regular (non-NIC) Patient	24.2	34.4	15.6	17.9	12.7	21.6
Male	26.0	30.1	17.4	19.7	14.4	22.6
Female	22.1	40.7	13.7	15.8	11.6	20.4
II. Average Stay for a NIC Patient	2.4	2.5	2.6	2.1	2.1	2.3
Male	2.4	2.3	2.3	2.2	2.0	2.2
Female	2.4	3.0	3.1	2.0	2.2	2.5

[a]January–April only.

Table 2–4
Number of Patients by Age Groups

	1969	*1970*	*1971*	*1972*	*1973*[a]	*1969–1973*
14–19	10	10	5	8	0	33 (5%)
20–24	14	21	16	17	4	72 (11%)
25–34	10	24	31	24	15	104 (16%)
35–50	37	33	45	52	20	187 (28%)
51–63	40	22	39	45	18	164 (25%)
64+	22	15	31	23	13	104 (16%)
Totals	133	125	167	169	70	664 (100%)

[a]January–April only.

Table 2–5
Number of Admissions by Patient Type and Sex

	Male	*Female*	*Totals*
Total Number of Admissions (all categories)	370 (55.7%)	294 (44.3%)	664 (100%)
I. Number of Regular (non-NIC) Admissions	255 (53%)	226 (47%)	481(100%)
II. Number of NIC Admissions	112 (62%)	68 (38%)	180 (100%)

Table 2–6
Number of Patients by Sex

	1969	*1970*	*1971*	*1972*	*1973*[a]	*1969–1973*
Number of Patients (all types)	133	125	167	169	70	664
Male	72	81	90	94	33	370
Female	61	44	77	75	37	294
I. Number of Regular (non-NIC) Patients	117	92	114	116	42	481
Male	61	37	59	64	16	255
Female	56	55	55	52	26	226
II. Number of NIC Patients	13	33	53	53	28	180
Male	8	26	31	30	17	112
Female	5	7	22	23	11	68

[a]January–April only.

board. Generally speaking, once the patient did leave the rehabilitation unit, there was little follow-up unless the patient had to return to the outpatient department for physical therapy.

The Rehabilitation Team

There are many and various roles to fill on a rehabilitation unit, and the complexity of these roles is increased by their relative importance to and effect upon the rehabilitation of the patient [17]. Rehabilitation in fact is a unique program in medical practice because it requires such a wide spectrum of input from supporting specialists; it is truly an interdisciplinary effort. Specialized physicians such as neurosurgeons, orthopedists, and physiatrists are, of course, required, but rehabilitation is most importantly a field in which nonphysician therapists are essential. Both the physical therapist and the occupational therapist are necessary to the practical integration of the patient into his community. Social workers, chaplains, and psychiatrists are called upon as guides to social and spiritual reintegration for the disabled patient. A dietary specialist must help the patient adapt to the particular diet he will need to sustain generally limited bodily functioning. Nurses, although they are not always trained in the field of rehabilitation [21], must attend the daily physical needs of the patient and inform others of any change in behavior or symptoms. In an auxiliary role, aides, orderlies, and assistants offer support to nursing and therapy staff by providing nontechnical patient services. Finally, there is the maintenance staff, those who clean and maintain the patient quarters and who, because of their intimate contact with the disabled, often develop close associations with them.

Recruiting the Staff Members

The Ward Director. As the leader of this new unit, the ward director was responsible for coordinating the various team members. He was to serve as liaison with hospital administration and with all other medical departments. Part of his task was to set medical policy for the unit, and he had ultimate supervision over and responsibility for all admission and treatment decisions. It was his job to supervise the treatment of each of the patients, to conduct a training program for residents and medical students, and to instruct the staff in the techniques of rehabilitation and of physical medicine. Finally, he was to be the representative for the hospital and the unit in all interactions with the community. One important qualification to the director's authority, one whose ramifications will be seen later on, was that the director did not have autonomous power to hire and fire his staff.

The person selected to fill the leadership role was a physiatrist. Head of the Division of Physical Medicine and Rehabilitation Department, his selection was particularly appropriate because it would enable him to teach rehabilitation on an inpatient basis while, at the same time, acting as teaching and administrative head of the new division. A man who had already achieved a reputation for professional excellence, kindness, and nonintrusiveness, he was regularly consulted by many staff and faculty at the hospital whenever they had a physical problem relating to his specialty because they felt that he was conservative, had good judgment, and would not intervene too rapidly. He was considered neither ruthless nor vindictive. His basic philosophical approach was that people would be cooperative and do their best if left to themselves.

Experts in the field of physical medicine and rehabilitation considered this ward director to be a pioneer in the field, not so much because of his research contribution as because he had been a leader for a long time and was considered highly competent both in the university and in the field of physical medicine and rehabilitation, generally. From a technical viewpoint, there was no question about his ability to direct such a unit.

For this man, the establishment of the ward was a dream finally realized. He had long recognized the need for a rehabilitation center, a place where patients with physical disabilities could be brought together and treated by a properly trained staff who were motivated for rehabilitation. He had conducted a campaign for just such a unit with hospital administrators and department chairpersons for many years. When the space became available, he was finally granted his wish.

The added prominence the new unit would bring to himself and his field were also important to the director. He felt he would no longer be as subordinate as he had been to other specialists; he would have his own territory with his own definitions. Ultimately, he wanted to separate from orthopedics, to make his specialty more autonomous and less dependent on other fields. With the inception of the unit, he visualized the possibility of forming an important and admired model that would provide both his field and himself with a greater measure of status and national respect.

The director soon discovered, however, that the problems of starting were as nothing compared with the complexities of running such a unit. The problems did not seem to be hierarchical, in the sense of some being more important than others, but rather seemed to have the quality of a carousel—the same problems kept coming around over and over and over again. Except for a change of label, these could have been the problems that existed when the ward was a psychiatric unit. The patients he was admitting were not "right." They either did not belong on a rehabilitation unit, or they were there for evaluation only, or there were too many quadriplegics and paraplegics, causing a work overload for the nursing staff. He had to keep the beds filled or risk the loss of staff, if not of the unit itself; and yet how was he to keep the ward filled if only ideal patients were to be admitted, and an ideal variety of those? There was no large pool of such patients waiting for admission to a unit that required that they pay for the treatment, themselves.

If he was often unhappy with the quality of his staff, the staff were often equally unhappy with the director. Many of the workers felt that he was not strong, not aggressive enough to run such a unit successfully. His perhaps naive attitude that people would naturally do their best allowed for much deviance that a more clearly delineated and controlled structure would not have permitted. A strictly defined system was needed to run this unit, and such a system was not imposed and did not emerge. Many of the staff saw the director as too patient-oriented and, perhaps reinforcing this sentiment or perhaps not, the patients almost unanimously saw the director as very concerned and involved with their rehabilitation progress.

The optimism with which the venture was begun, the wishful thinking that filled the gaps in planning and staffing slowly faded, and the director saw his dream become a tangled web of problems that no amount of patience, prayer, or willpower was going to be able to unravel.

The Head Nurse. While the director of the unit had worked many years in the field of rehabilitation, the head nurse had no previous experience or training in rehabilitation whatsoever. Availability and seniority formed the primary basis for her selection. She was hired within the organization, where she had been a head nurse on a medical unit quite different from the rehabilitation unit in its structure, its rapid turnover of patients, and its task orientation.

As the chief administrative officer of the unit, the head nurse was responsible for the unit's minute-to-minute, hour-to-hour, day-to-day operation. She supervised all aspects of patient care, making sure that patients had food, that they were changed, that they received medication, and were transported to and from the areas to which they needed to go for X-rays, physical therapy, and laboratory examinations. She coordinated the activities of the various physicians; and she talked to family members and explained to them how the patient was doing, when the patient could be visited, what progress had been made, and what the physician who was not present might have said. The head nurse sat at the top of the pyramid where the communication of written and oral information began.

Although she was the major administrator on the unit and had many staff members working under her, she was by no means autonomous in her authority, however. As the nurses, LVNs, aides, technicians, and even ward clerks were subject to her direction, so she herself was answerable to many others. The medical director of the unit was her boss. The entire supervising nursing structure oversaw her activities and could direct her to make changes. Also, the patient's physician and the resident in charge of the patient could make alterations in the treatment regimen.

It is essential to the effective operation of a head nurse that those members of the team whose activities she coordinates and who are not directly under her supervision recognize her authority to coordinate. If they do not, then there are serious problems. The head nurse can manage insubordination or recalcitrance from those underneath her only if those above give her support; and her superiors can support her only if they think she is right. Once right and wrong enter the picture (and they always do), the need for arbitration also enters. Because there often are conflicts of interest and conflicts of values about what is right, there must be some sort of negotiating mechanism. If the negotiating mechanism breaks down, a dynamic process of disintegration can occur, the head nurse becoming demoralized, depressed, angry, and diminished in the eyes of those she must command. This is, in fact, what happened on the rehabilitation unit.

The head nurse was dissatisfied with almost every aspect of the unit. She was upset with the leaders of the unit, feeling they did not support her, and her greatest complaint was that they themselves were afraid to make decisions. She was frustrated by what she felt was the incompetence of some of her nursing staff and the slight control she could exercise over them. She felt that they did not help her in making decisions and forced her to bear the brunt of being the authority figure. (It is interesting that the psychiatric head nurses had made the same complaints.)

The staff and patients were equally conflicted about the head nurse. Some felt her to be highly competent and concerned; others felt her to be too authoritarian and insistent on her own way of doing things, too concerned with administrative details and the letter rather than the spirit of the unit laws.

Particularly destructive was the conflict between the director and the head nurse. He had looked to her for the kind of leadership that would organize and structure the unit as a therapeutic reality. He had hoped she would infuse it with a spirit that would convert it from a set of procedures into a vital, enthusiastic, inspired center for repairing the spirit and the flesh of broken human beings. She had expected the same of him. Neither was satisfied with the other.

Physical Therapists. The physical therapists, selected from the ward director's department and experienced in their area on both an inpatient and outpatient basis, filled a key position in the rehabilitation unit. It was the physical therapist who performed most of the actual exercises with the patient and whose goal it was to achieve the patient's physical rehabilitation. The patient's day was, in fact, planned around the physical therapist and was supposed to be designed so that the patient would receive maximum benefit from the therapist's limited five-days-a-week presence.

Unlike the nurses, aides, orderlies, and maintenance staff, the physical therapists worked on a rotation schedule, staying with the rehabilitation unit for six to eight weeks and then returning to the physical-therapy department. Rotation of the physical therapists arose, in part, because the rehabilitation unit was considered the ideal or model unit, and thus most of the physical therapists preferred assignment to it. The prospect of working on a truly interdisciplinary team was enticing. Usually physical therapists operated on the various hospital floors or in the outpatient physical-therapy setting and had relatively little exchange with other members of the health-care team. They seldom dealt with the physician except through the orders that he or she wrote. They seldom conversed with the nurses on the floor. They had little contact with the families of the patient. In fact, they were not members of an integrated team but were doing an individual, assigned task, such as teaching the patient to walk on crutches or helping him acquire eating skills or exercising weakened muscles. Initially, they thought that working on the inpatient service would be a more gratifying, more exciting experience and would offer greater opportunity for the kind of extended care that each professional group believes its clients or patients need. Thus, the physical therapists' desire to work on the rehabilitation unit reflected fulfillment of their dreams—the possibility of working as members of a health-care team, of relating to other professionals, of participating in planning goals, and of meeting with families. This seemed the ideal way to treat patients, and they wanted to participate in it. By rotating the staff, each would be able to work in this highly valued setting.

But with rotation also came difficulties. Had one or two physical therapists been assigned permanently to the new inpatient service, they might have come more under the influence of the unit's authority. As it was, they remained essentially under the wing of the physical-therapy department, only tangentially (and then only temporarily) allied to the rehabilitation unit.

The quality also fluctuated. Some of the therapists were outstanding and were recognized as great therapists by the director, other physicians, their peers, the nursing staff, and ultimately by the patients themselves. Others were felt to be inadequate to the task of caring for and treating a helpless, disabled patient. In a way, the rehabilitation unit became a fishbowl for the physical therapists, who previously had been able to avoid scrutiny because their work had been done on one of the wards or in the privacy of a cubicle in the outpatient physical-therapy section. On the rehabilitation unit, however, the physical therapist was observed closely by every single member of the staff, and patients who had been on the ward for some time could compare one therapist with another.

About one physical therapist in particular, the director received many complaints from staff, patients, parents of patients, and other physicians. Undoubtedly intelligent and competent, this therapist was either psychologically unequipped to care for patients or she had no interest in doing so, and there were no provisions for relieving the ward of a staff member whose failure could have such a costly effect on the patients. But even when the incoming therapist was highly talented, the change in routine that took place with each new therapist was difficult for many patients. Signs of depression and acting-out behavior would appear whenever a good therapist was about to leave the ward. This presented a typical on-the-one-hand, on-the-other-hand dilemma for which there seemed to be no solution satisfactory to all concerned. The director could not bring himself to sacrifice the opportunity for many physical therapists to gain experience working on the ward, and so rotation continued.

Ironically, as it became apparent that the inpatient unit might not live up to the expectations of the staff, rotation became desirable because assignment to the unit was less sought after than assignment to the outpatient physical-therapy service or to work on the hospital floors. While the therapists had once wanted to be part of an interdisciplinary team, it now became important for them to remain in touch with their own colleagues for communication and support. Finally, when there were indications that the unit might not survive, the physical therapists saw assignment to it as a duty, a turn they had to take, a cleanup operation.

The Core Service Staff. The core staff included the people most directly in touch with and responsible for the daily needs of the patients and the ward. Although this was a highly specialized unit, the nurses and supporting staff were recruited from the rest of the hospital, because the work was not considered essentially different from that in the general hospital. There was an acute shortage of nurses at that time, making it necessary for the director to hire inexperienced nurses who had not worked directly with disabled persons before and had to learn the techniques for treating such patients and for interacting with other members of the unit.

As with the physical therapists, some of the nurses were considered excellent and others ineffective. Some were flexible and able in a pleasant way to get patients to do the things that would help them to recover, and some were seen as too strict or too firm and, as a result, patients (to their own detriment) resisted the staff's efforts to help them.

Evaluation of the nurses was, in fact, one of the areas of conflict between the director and the head nurse, for the nurses whom he considered to be most outstanding were often precisely the ones she regarded as unsuitable. For example, the director described one nurse as "excellent," because her concern for patients was her first priority and everything else came second. The head nurse, however, saw this same nurse as highly unsuitable because she did not attend to her paperwork or to the administrative requirements of the hospital, burdening the other nurses with her tasks so that they were less able to provide for the patients' needs.

There were three nurse and supporting staff shifts that differed markedly in the type of care provided and in the relation of staff members to patients. The day shift was at the center of the unit's hustle and bustle, seeing that the patients were where they were supposed to be and doing what they were supposed to do, interacting with other members of the unit and with visitors, and, in general, on the move. Their relationships with the patients tended to be joking and casual, as there was little time for more intimate involvement. The evening staff, on the other hand, often developed closer relationships with the patients. The ward had calmed down, most of the people were gone, and the patients needed company as well as physical care. A warm, friendly voice was then a great asset. By the time the night shift came on, the ward was silent, most of the patients having already gone to bed. The night shift had virtually no contact with day personnel; their main duty was to turn patients regularly and to force them to drink fluids; and the isolation these staff members felt from the rest of the ward was sometimes a problem.

Because the evening and night shifts were not exposed to view as the day staff was, and because the supporting staff essentially selected itself for duty on the ward, another hazard existed. When work involves intimate contact with those who are disabled and physically helpless, there is always the risk of exploitation and sadistic behavior. It is possible and, in fact, probable that some of the self-selected workers found the ward an avenue for "acting out" their own frustrations or psychopathology.

The Specialty Therapist. In any rehabilitation unit the specialty therapist would have been considered a key member. If it was the role of the nurse to maintain basic care functions, and if it was the role of the physical therapist to develop physical range and strength, then it was the role of this staff member to develop what one might call the civilized skills. It was this person's responsibility to make it possible for the patient to care for himself and to begin the task of contributing productively to society. One of the most unfortunate and discouraging problems the ward experienced centered around the specialty therapist.

The director's trouble with the specialty therapist had begun many years earlier, when he had at one time tried to discharge the person but had been defeated in this effort through a grievance procedure. When the opportunity came to start the rehabilitation unit and there were no funds available to hire a second therapist, the director decided that it would be more prudent to accept the situation as it was rather than indicate to the administration that there was no point in making this large investment on a unit unless one could staff the ward with the kinds of people who would make it function effectively. The result was predictable; if the staff members rallied together on no other point, they were unanimous in their criticism of the specialty therapist. It was felt that she had little ability to interest the patients in what she was trying to teach. It was also felt that she did not really work to interest the patients and that she was not persistent in urging patients to try if once they indicated to her that they were not fully appreciative of her efforts or if they appeared unmotivated.

If there was one scapegoat on the ward, it was this woman, and it is possible that the frustration the director and others felt was symbolic. The specialty therapist represented organizational immobilization. To each staff member, she occasioned the feeling that "if only we could have different people, this place would function well." The frustration felt because unintegrated members could not be fired acted as a crippling force throughout the life of the unit.

Other Members of the Staff. In addition to those already described, there were numerous part-time and occasional workers on the unit. These included social workers, dieticians, chaplains, students, and orthopedic residents. It was the social worker's job to study the patient's resources and social network. Since, in order to remain on the unit, the patient would have to be supported by some outside agency, his family, a private insurance carrier, or the community, it was the social worker's business to assess this network and to mobilize all the resources possible to facilitate the patient's recovery. It was also the social worker's responsibility to investigate future occupations in which the patient might be interested and to serve as liaison between the family and the staff, between the community and the staff, and between the community and the family. As with the physical therapists and the nurses, the social worker's success on the unit varied with the personality, professional competence, and interest of the individual. The fact that a social worker could be assigned (and, indeed, was assigned) without the approval of or any consultation with the director of the unit indicated severe communication problems between the university administration and the unit administration, communication problems that could also be seen in the residents who worked on the unit.

None of the residents planned to make physical medicine and rehabilitation a specialty or subspecialty. Surgery was the high-status activity in their training programs, and anyone who demonstrated special interest in physical medicine and rehabilitation lost status with his peers and superiors. As duty on the unit was a part-time assignment, the resident was expected to learn all that he could while on the ward, but his loyalties and identification remained with his primary group of orthopedic residents and faculty. Ironically, much of an orthopedist's professional work is not surgical but is closely related to the evaluations and procedures a resident would learn while on the rehabilitation unit. Evaluating for rehabilitation potential, designing complex rehabilitation programs, and predicting the probability of success of rehabilitation efforts–these are all very much a part of an orthopedist's job, but the interest shown by the residents while on the unit was slight.

The director and the head nurse were united in their dissatisfaction with most of the residents, who seemed to see the assignment as a chore, as part of the price they had to pay for staying in their residency. They were difficult to find and frequently did not respond to calls as promptly as was wished. When they did come, the staff sensed that they were uninterested in what was going on and saw the staff's request for orders or care or participation as burdensome. They seemed generally clumsy in relating to patients with profound physical disturbances and, although they seemed quite able to deal with acute crisis situations, they were unable to interact successfully with a patient whose long-term prognosis was poor.

This brief description of the team members suggests the complex interaction necessary for a unit such as this one to succeed, and the serious problems that arise when all members of the team do not share a compatible set of values, experiences, and goals.

The least amount of time spent at the unit was by the physician. Whether psychiatrist or physiatrist or orthopedist, he spent probably no more than one or two hours a day on the unit. In some ways he was the visiting dignitary, the inspector general. He came, he looked, he ordered, he assuaged, and he left. This person, who spent the least amount of time on the unit, was the patient's greatest source of power. It was only through him that the patient could change his environment in a substantial way. Change in treatment regimen and increase or decrease in participation in other activities on the unit were, by and large, under the control of the physician. Although the patient was actually free to leave the hospital whenever he wanted, either by telling the physician that he wanted to leave and obtaining the physician's consent or by leaving against medical advice, the patient seldom did either. He negotiated with his physician, first for passes and later for discharge; or the negotiations might be reversed, with the physician pushing for more outside activities, more separation from the hospital, less dependence on the residential treatment center. Whatever his role with any particular patient, the physician was a key man on the team, and his sorcererlike presence (now you see him, now you don't) along with his lack of interaction with the rest of the staff left the unit vulnerable to cross-messages (the physician telling the patient one thing, the staff telling him another), morale problems, and patient dissatisfaction.

Similarly, the consulting psychiatrist often was thought to be less involved in the unit than was wished. Granting that unreasonable hopes sometimes are laid upon psychiatrists and that no psychiatrist could single-handedly have solved all of the unit's difficulties, still, a full-time psychiatrist could have played a very important role in the dynamics of the unit. Many of the staff strongly felt the need for group counseling, help in figuring out how to approach a patient, how to understand a patient's particular reactions to any given situation, how to manage the staff's own feelings about or reactions to a patient. The psychiatrist could have been a kind of safety valve for tension, a mediator between patients and staff and staff and staff. While the psychiatrist was available on a consulting basis, many of the team members felt that this was not enough. It was also felt by many staff members that a full-time psychiatrist should have been part of the rehabilitation team just to see the patients on a regular basis. That a rehabilitation patient will have emotional problems related to his disability almost goes without saying, and regular psychiatric therapy could have had a highly beneficial effect on the patients' emotional adjustment. As it was, therapy occurred intermittently or when the patient specifically requested it, and inasmuch as the psychiatrist assigned was not always the same, the therapy could not be considered continuous.

These problems and their consequences will be discussed more fully in later sections on patient-staff and staff-staff interactions.

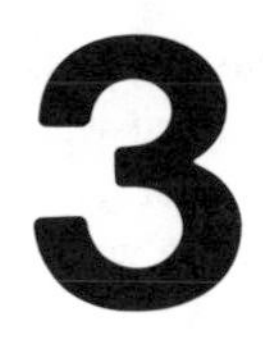

Roles, Values, and Culture

For a number of reasons, people are reluctant to define roles, whether in the family or in the university or in a work situation. There is a prevailing feeling that role definition is dangerous, that it will restrict creativity and limit freedom, that it is fascistic, or that it represents a kind of compulsivity that leads to rigid, static environments. Because of reluctance to define roles for themselves or to be seen as strict role definers of others, those involved in the evaluation of organizations seldom approach the role-fulfillment problem in any but a very general way. Needless to say, such an approach to roles will create an atmosphere in which there is very little role correction, and roles will evolve in a haphazard rather than a systematic way.

Let us posit a working rule: When people have ill- or loosely defined roles, they tend in the direction of the most pleasant activity for themselves. Thus, in a hospital, when roles are loosely defined, personnel will move in the direction of nontouching; that is, they will move away from interaction with patients and toward interaction with each other. Or, when many and various roles are to be filled by one person and those roles are casually defined, that person usually will emphasize those roles that are highest status or most personally satisfying and will subordinate those that are more troublesome, time-consuming, or menial. The ideal professional would, of course, understand perfectly all the elements that composed his role and would regulate himself so that all functions were satisfactorily fulfilled. However, to ask a mere human being to achieve such a goal without a clearly defined set of rules and expectations would be to ask him to stop being human. Therefore, at the risk of being called fascistic or compulsive, we will insist that roles, in order to be optimally fulfilled, must be well defined from the outset. If each person wants to conduct the concert and no one wants to play the way the conductor directs him to play, it is not likely that the orchestra will perform successfully. If, however, each person sticks to his own particular instrument, which he is well qualified to play, and follows the conductor's directions, then the orchestra will create what it was meant to create—music.

Perhaps we can further illuminate our conception of a good professional by analogy with a waiter in a top-notch restaurant. The waiter has a very clear notion of what his job is. He serves other people, and he does not feel that serving other people diminishes him in any way. In other words, if he has to take some offensive treatment from someone, he takes it as part of his job. He might afterwards complain, but basically he says, "No, sir," or "Yes, sir," within the limits of his work role. Now, if the customer asks him to run out and buy him a pack of cigarettes across the street, the waiter might well say, "My job ends at the door. I don't go beyond there. Sorry, but I won't be able to do that for you, sir." But within his defined role, the waiter fulfills his obligations to serve.

The example of the waiter holds true for all professionals. In order to protect the professional from his own feelings, from his own reactions, roles must be clearly defined. The good waiter does not become indignant or vindictive when a customer tells him, "I don't like what you serve." He does not take it personally, and neither should a health professional. This does not mean that the professional has to deny his own feelings about liking some people or disliking others, but that these feelings should have as little influence on his professional relationship with the patient or other staff person as possible. Role definitions in this context are the antithesis of enslavement. Instead, they free the worker from his own reactions so that he can effectively do his job.

There are any number of ways to define roles. Perhaps the strictest adherence to role definitions can be seen in those unions whose members are absolutely forbidden to infringe upon the roles of other workers. For instance, in the movie industry a certain type of electrician or stagehand might have to be hired for an extended period of time to do one single task. While he is waiting to do his particular job, he will stand around, observe others working, read, or do whatever he chooses. Such a role pattern will produce a smile or anger depending upon whether or not the one observing the pattern is also paying for it. However, should an oversight occur and the particular specialist not be hired, rather than cross role boundaries the whole crew will stop working as soon as they come to the part of the job the missing specialist should do. There are many such restrictions in the crafts unions, and by now they are generally accepted, provoking little of the outrage they once occasioned.

Such strict definitions are not generally characteristic of the medical field. No one in a medical setting is supposed to sit around for eight hours a day in order to turn one valve or to handle one kind of operation. It is generally expected that whatever a medical or health professional is doing in a hospital setting will require all of his working time. If all of his time is not occupied, then it is assumed that fewer persons are needed for the type of job or that the job itself might not be necessary and should be contracted out. Thus, special nurses are not kept waiting in the hospital so that they will be available when a patient requires full-time care. They are called in only when they are actually needed.

Because time-use is an important criterion for defending the necessity of a health professional's job, it becomes difficult to define role boundaries too strictly. The health professional may not be able to use all of the time for which he is being paid unless he moves into another person's role, does more than is considered to be within the boundaries of his particular job, or is unusually creative and can develop new aspects of his role without invading someone else's territory. Or, as is seen quite often in hospital settings and as was a common occurrence on the rehabilitation ward, the worker could try to get someone else to take time off with him. A casual conversation, a cup of coffee, a party to be planned—these were only the most common in an endless list of diversions. Such diversions did not tend to occur as single incidents on the ward; they happened again and again as the persons involved tested each other, became more intimate, and found the diversionary measures mutually satisfying. The dangers inherent in this sort of "goofing off" syndrome are obvious and sometimes fatal.

When designing a unit and prescribing roles, those in authority must plan how time is going to be utilized, and they must particularly consider potential "dead time." If this is not taken into account, one risks losing not only the services of the person whose abilities are not needed at the moment but also the services of many others who are needed. Also, if one worker's role includes a prolonged period of "dead time," as in the example we described of the stagehand, then a morale problem is created. How can one staff member work full time, doing everything that needs to be done, working without more than an ordinary coffee break or half-hour lunch, while another staff person is doing almost nothing, sitting around reading, watching television, talking to patients, or knitting? It is easy to underestimate this as a morale factor, and we often prefer to ignore it because of the difficulty of planning for "dead time" in any kind of setting; however, as observation and interviews with the staff on the rehabilitation unit made clear, it is a problem that cannot be ignored if a unit is to operate effectively.

On this unit, there was no planning for "dead time." In fact, there was no planning for "live time," either. There was some assignment of tasks, and these were role specific. For instance, the physical therapist had tasks connected with physical therapy but not with passing out medications or taking temperatures or blood pressures, and the orderlies performed maintenance roles but did not officially advise a patient concerning his insurance problems. The nurses, however, had a broader role definition, and there was no reason why a nurse should not help a patient in a general way with some of his physical therapy even though the finer aspects were left to the physical therapist. But because the responsibilities included in each worker's role were not carefully delineated, the option of helping out or not helping out was left mainly to the discretion of the team member involved.

Roles represent an abstract that can be talked about in specific terms. An operational definition of role would describe accurately what one does with one's time, and how one uses a given period of time, such as the eight hours a day spent at work. The specific setting must also be considered in any practical definition of role. It is not enough to say, for example, that someone is a nurse. The nurse role cannot be understood unless we know what things this particular nurse does and exactly how the time is spent. Nurses, doctors, nurses' aides, and ward clerks often do the same kinds of things. We could not tell the difference between them simply by observing one given piece of behavior or one given activity. But if we know the distribution of activity, how the different people spend their time on the average, then we can talk about the nurse's role in a specific setting or the doctor's role on a specific unit rather than a nurse's or doctor's role in general.

The need to be specific when defining roles is particularly applicable to the rehabilitation unit, for while many acute-care units require the same sorts of services from their team members, the rehabilitation unit's definition of a worker's role often differs markedly from that of other units. An obvious example of this is in the concept of nurse. According to the head nurse on the rehabilitation unit, a nurse is usually seen as one who "takes care of" or "does for" a patient. An incoming patient finds himself reduced to a child in the hospital setting. He is stripped of his clothes, told to put on a robe, and given orders to do this or do that. In the rehabilitation ward, however, the patient does for himself because he is being trained to return to a normal life. The nurse's role on this ward, then, becomes as much involved with insisting on a patient's independence as it is involved with caring for the patient in those areas where he cannot be independent.

A second distinction that must be made when defining job roles is the difference between the prescriptive role and the evolved one. An official job description may have little in common with the job itself, and the role often evolves as a compromise between the supervisor's dictation of the job's necessities and the worker's day-to-day study of what is needed and what is palatable. Consider, for example, the case of a newly hired staff nurse. On the day she starts her job on the ward, she begins to follow the various written prescriptions. In order to fulfill the immediate requirements of the job, however, she will begin to make a minute-by-minute analysis of the job requirements, adapting her activities as she deems necessary. Consequently, her role functions eventually may differ from the expectations of the head nurse or other staff members. The staff nurse might discover as a result of her evaluation of the actual requirements of the job that she does not like the job or is not suited to it. She must then either remake the role, or she must leave. If the head nurse does not approve of the way the staff nurse is remaking her role, the staff nurse will be corrected and then she must adapt to the correction. The head nurse might say, "No, you have to do more of this and less of that." The staff nurse then changes her activities, though not exactly as directed. Eventually, as this procedure is repeated again and again, a stable role will evolve.

A third way in which roles are influenced, if not determined, comes as a result of pressures applied by other staff members. A doctor, a physical therapist, and a custodian, for example, will have different expectations of what a nurse's role should be, and they will communicate these expectations in subtle or overt ways. The nurse must then either incorporate these views into her own conception of her role, or she must be proof against the impractical or wrongly directed expectations of the other team members. One of the complaints registered by the head nurse on the rehabilitation ward was that no one would share the authority role with her. None of the nursing staff ever wanted to say "no" to a patient, so all questions were referred to the head nurse. For instance, one of the aides wanted to wash a patient's hair during a period that was a work time for the patient. All parties knew that this was not allowed, but the burden of refusal was still put upon the head nurse. No one else would take the responsibility of verbalizing what they all knew to be a rule. Peer, superior, and subordinate pressures are perhaps the most potentially destructive of the influences that determine roles because they, in effect, manipulate the staff member into taking on responsibilities that are inappropriate or into carrying alone a burden that should be shared. This is one of the areas in which a clearly delineated definition of role can greatly alleviate the problem.

Roles on the Rehabilitation Unit

As a medical organization is an intricate web whose every fiber is a potential source of strength and reinforcement or of weakness, contamination, and disruption, a systems analysis can be an important aid in unwinding the fibers of this interlaced structure [27]. Thus, through a systems analysis, we can see the various types of stratification in a medical unit, stratification that helps to determine roles and role models.

Socioeconomic class lines form one basis of stratification on a medical unit; that is, members at the leadership level generally come from higher socioeconomic classes than those at the service level. Power and seniority are another basis of stratification; professional specialization constitutes yet a third. Certain activities and areas of authority usually are reserved for specialty groups. In some medical practices one person, a general practitioner, for instance, is permitted to conduct all the diagnostic and therapeutic treatments, but this rarely is the case in a specialized medical unit. Written and unwritten rules govern not only who is to do what procedures but how they are to be performed and in what manner they are to be carried out. Any given role on a medical unit will combine a number of often conflicting types of stratification, and unless clear definitions exist that delineate the rights, responsibilities, and authorities of a role, confusion almost inevitably will arise as to who should do what and when. For example, a role may involve high power but low seniority, and unless specific rules describe each role's responsibilities, a conflict may occur when the member with high power but low seniority interacts with a staff member whose power is lower but whose seniority is high.

Within this rehabilitation unit, specific titles were used to designate the roles of the various staff members, but beyond these titles, the staff themselves developed their roles or operational procedures for best handling the time they spent on the ward. We found four types of staff role: the *leadership role*, which was assumed sometimes by the director, sometimes by the head nurse, and, toward the end of the unit's life, by the nursing service outside the ward; the *subleadership role*, which was filled by the assisting nurses, the therapists, and the social worker; the *service role*, which was given to the aides, hospital assistants, orderlies, and maintenance crew; and the *consultant role*, which was assumed by those staff (the administrator, the physicians, the psychiatrist, and the chaplains) who did not work full-time on the ward but who provided consultant services. The consultant's role sometimes entailed leadership and sometimes subleadership responsibilities. For example, when an outside physician referred a patient to the ward, he acted in a leadership capacity, but the psychiatrist's weekly visits to the ward, or the administrator's procurement of a television set or dining-room table, would fall into the subleadership category.

The amount of time spent on the unit had an important effect on how well each staff member could fill his role, and those in the highest leadership positions were often those who spent the least amount of time on the ward (see figure 3-1).

The Leadership Role

Most important to the guidance of this rehabilitation unit was the role of the leader. Besides the authority specifically granted to him, the leader's power depended on his personal relationships with his staff and on his ability to enforce his rulings. Since, as noted earlier, the leader was not given the authority to hire and fire, to promote and demote, he could enforce his dictates only if most of the participants on the unit agreed that the leader had the right to issue directives, that the subordinates had the obligation to obey the rules, and that disobedience would bring not only rightful vengeance from above but also disapproval and ostracism by peers and subordinates. It would be an understatement to say that this is a big "if." The leader who is unaware of these qualifications to his power may make a big splash, but he will slowly drown in a sea of his subordinates' resistance and his superiors' temporizing comments and warnings.

The quality and quantity of leadership is an issue in all institutions and in their subunits. Leaders cannot help but arouse strong feelings in their subordinates, even as parents arouse strong feelings in their children, and subordinates pass judgment on their leaders much as children do on their parents. In most discussions of leadership roles and problems, the focus is on the leader's decision-making process, his actions, and the response of his subordinates in

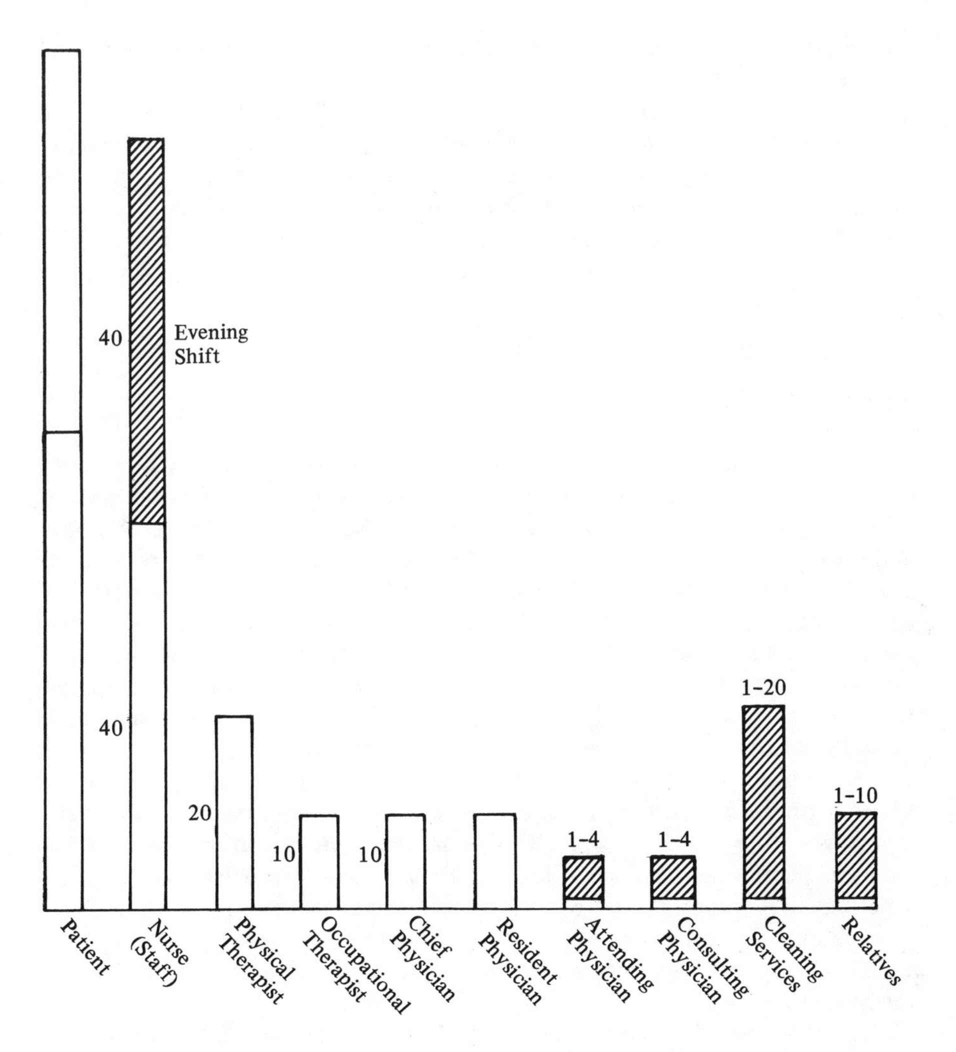

Figure 3-1. Time Spent in Rehabilitation Unit (hours per week) by Role Designation

action and in feeling. Seldom are the leader's problems or his feelings and judgments considered. While our ideal professional would never allow his feelings to interfere with his professional objectivity, in analyzing a system as small as the rehabilitation unit where relationships between team members were highly developed and sometimes intimate, we cannot ignore the leader as a vulnerable human being. Nor can we pass over the importance of the feedback channels from subordinate to leader and back to subordinate if we are to understand the field in which a leader's decisions are produced, enforced, and altered. Many of the problems faced by the ward director as leader of the rehabilitation unit were problems inherent in the leadership role itself, and because of their systemic importance, they will be discussed in greater detail in Chapter 8.

The head nurse also acted in a leadership capacity as the minute-to-minute authority on the unit. Because the actual extent of her authority was not specifically designated, she and the ward director were often in conflict about how far her power should reach and, as will also be discussed later, it was thought that the head nurse tried to usurp some of the authority that should have been the province of the ward director.

Subleadership Roles

Subleaders on the rehabilitation unit included physical and specialty therapists, social workers, assistant head nurses, and the supervising nurse who was in charge of the evening and night shifts. Ideally, their roles would be carefully defined by the leaders, and their authority would lie in carrying out the leader's directives. If the leader's directives are not explicit, however, or if they are not agreed upon by the subleaders, then we will find the subleaders taking either more or less responsibility and power upon themselves than their roles require. An example of this occurring on the rehabilitation unit can be seen in relation to the specialty therapist already described. Her role responsibilities should have extended far beyond the boundaries she actually chose to define.

A problem also occurred on the unit when there was conflict between leaders, either between the leaders and the subleaders or between the subleaders themselves. These conflicts would tend to be acted out in relationships with the patients. Stanton and Schwartz [28], in their studies of problems in a psychiatric unit, demonstrated that when patients became disturbed it often was not possible initially to determine the nature of their disturbance, but further study would disclose staff conflicts that were being acted out with the patients and by the patients.

On the rehabilitation ward, one of the continuing conflicts among staff members and between staff and patients centered around what the atmosphere of the unit should be, whether it should be permissive or restrictive. This conflict was acted out by the patients through their use of drugs and by the nurses, aides, and patients through some of the erotic and sadistic relationships that occurred. It is important to note that this acting out is *not* conscious. Neither patient nor staff person nor leader makes the conscious decision to do something destructive. The behavior is rationalized as therapeutic or as an expression of the rights of the actor, even though those rights have not been specifically granted.

Another example of acting out common on the ward occurred often as a result of a staff person's anger. The angry staff person might respond slowly to a patient's call, and the patient would note this and in turn respond uncooperatively toward the physical therapist. The physical therapist would talk to the nurse, who would rationalize her late response by indicating that the patient was too demanding. The physical therapist would then contribute by saying that the patient was also uncooperative. Neither would recognize that something occurring at the staff level had triggered all the patient's reactions.

Service Roles

Service workers, including aides, orderlies, and LVNs, formed a core group on the staff. Because far less of their time was devoted to paperwork or administrative problems than was that of other staff, they were available for more intense patient contact. They also had fewer defenses against closeness than did the professional staff. They were not concerned about their own status or socioeconomic background and therefore had nothing to lose by mixing with patients. Neither had they been trained to maintain a professional distance from a patient or to remain objective about his problems, as had the more rigorously schooled staff members. Their roles included administering to the basic needs of the patient in ambulation, cleaning, and maintenance of bodily function. Because they often saw the patient in pain, they were more frustrated than others when problems in patient care could not be resolved by the leaders and subleaders. They often had to witness a patient's misery, but they seldom could assuage it, and this sometimes would occasion a situation where the service worker would subvert the patient's therapy or the unit's rules by bringing the patient drugs or alcohol. This, of course, created tremendous conflicts between the service workers and the leaders and subleaders.

From an organizational standpoint, the service workers were removed from the leadership struggle. They were affected by but not involved in the power plays between leaders and subleaders. An undifferentiated group of helpers, they performed an enormous amount of assigned work without having any substantial role in determining treatment plans. Exactly how much work a service staff person did was far less dependent on his role definition than on his abilities, motivation, and involvement. The service worker who was bright, eager, kind, and personable, for example, preferred a variety of therapeutic functions along with his assigned role. The worker, on the other hand, who was just putting in time or who was unhappy on the ward often did very little.

Service workers, in particular the nursing personnel, often felt they were doing the work of the subleaders, such as that of the specialty therapist, in addition to their own tasks. One aide also felt that at times he had to assume the role of the psychiatrist, and this, in fact, led him to problems with one patient.

Twice I can remember being tense and upset. One patient was trying to find a psychiatrist and I tried to explain something to him that should have been explained by someone else. He wouldn't accept it and reported me to the director. He was a paraplegic, and he wasn't going to accept the idea that he was a paraplegic, and he didn't want to do the work. It was easy to see the conflict between him and his wife, and I think I mentioned it to him and said, "Well, in some cases, you know you'll be left behind and your wife will probably go out shopping." I think he took it another way. He thought that I was saying his wife was going to leave him. She did.

Whatever the right of the service person to act in a psychiatrist's role and whatever the motivations that actually lay behind this discussion about the patient's wife, this example clearly demonstrates both the intimacy that could arise between patients and service personnel and the therapeutic problems that could occur as a result of that intimacy. Whenever roles are loosely enough defined that an unqualified worker can assume the role which only a qualified worker should fill, the consequences can be highly destructive to the unit's goals.

Consultant Roles

A variety of consultants came onto the rehabilitation unit, and these differed markedly in their degree of contact and involvement with the unit. At one extreme were those consultants whose contact was very brief and limited in scope. These consultants would enter and exit, and practically the only mark they left would be a note in the records or a telephone call to the physician who had requested their services. Included among these consultants were ear-nose-and-throat specialists, eye specialists, and sometimes internists. Generally speaking, these consultants had very little impact on ward life. They specifically helped the patient or the referring physician, and they acted as reporters to other people on the effectiveness and atmosphere of the unit, but their roles were limited to these two functions.

At the other extreme were those consultants who became quite involved with the unit. These included the psychiatric consultant and the spiritual consultant, the chaplain. In order to perform their roles well, these team members had to work closely with the staff and with the patients' families. They often became involved in the operations of the unit and participated in staff conferences.

The consultant role could be a very helpful one to the health of the unit. Because he was not an integral part of the ward life and thus not enmeshed in the politics, interpersonal tensions, and gratifications of the unit, the consultant often was more objective in his evaluation of a patient's problems and the effectiveness of his treatment.

A consultant who had the skills (and this is an important qualification) was often able to help staff members communicate with patients or to relieve staff tension in working with a patient. Because he was relatively dispassionate, he often could recognize trouble spots between staff and patients and smooth over those problem areas by helping each to understand the general situation and the other person better. Sometimes a consultant could give quite specific or technical advice for a patient's treatment. One consultant on the ward, for example, noticed that a patient tended to be sleepy at a certain time of the day because of the medications he was taking, and therefore advised against trying to engage him in certain activities during that time. The consultant would also take into account the patient's psychological, social, religious, and cultural background and advise treatment accordingly. He might thus be able to suggest a better way to approach a situation in order to achieve the agreed-upon goals.

Consultants, on the other hand, could also be a source of problems and dissatisfaction. Like the outside observer in any situation, it was easy for the consultant to come onto the unit, immediately see all of its problems, and know precisely how to solve them. He knew what the other physicians were doing wrong, what the family was doing wrong; in effect, he understood the whole situation. Some consultants thought they knew how to cure all the problems and that the way to cure them was simply for patients and staff to "shape up" and behave correctly.

There are several dangers in having a consultant come in and know too much too soon. First, if the consultant's criticisms reach the patient's ears, as they so often do, the patient can become dissatisfied or he can become concerned about whether he is getting the quality of care he needs.

Second, the consultant's reactions and perceptions can be disruptive to staff relations. Some staff persons, especially those who agree with the consultant, come to feel overly justified in their own diagnoses; others may feel blamed and unfairly judged if they disagree with him. In this situation, the consultant becomes a destructive rather than an integrative force on the unit.

Unfortunately, many consultants are not aware that there are both positive and negative implications to their roles, and they rush in to give advice without thinking that the responsibility for the consequences of that advice will fall on another. Advice that cannot practically be implemented can have only a destructive wish-denial effect on the patients and staff, and advice that is not carefully considered can bring in its wake a whole new set of problems that might not have emerged were it not for the advice. A consultant, who can be a very powerful force for change on a unit, must be wary of simple solutions. In other words, he must at all times be cognizant of his potential power.

Values

First, we must ask what we mean by the term "value." One definition [29] is that value is "an abstract concept, often merely implicit, that defines for an individual or for a social unit what ends or means to an end are desirable" (p. 577). Usually, individuals do not create their own idiosyncratic values but, rather, slowly incorporate society's values into their own working theories. As values tend to find their strength in the unity of the group adhering to them, any opposition to accepted values from within a group can cause severe conflicts. Such conflicts were clearly manifested on the rehabilitation ward.

A complication that arises in any attempt to analyze a group's values is that the values are not absolute; they fluctuate depending upon the role a person is assuming at the time. One of the important contributions of the late Eric Berne was his recognition that each individual possesses three different ego states: a parent ego, an adult ego, and a child ego [30]. This concept forms the basis of his transactional model of interpersonal relationships, and while Berne's specific elaboration may be questioned, few would deny its underlying validity. If we watch a person talking to his superior and then to his subordinate, we can quickly see how the person changes the way he behaves, adapting his role to fit the nature of his relationship with each person.

This same phenomenon appears in relation to values, attitudes, expectations, and norms. We might naively expect that a person's values will be consistent, that a nurse, for example, will have the same attitudes, values, and expectations when she is a patient as when she is a nurse; or that a patient will hold the same attitudes and values he held before becoming a patient. In fact, all of these change, and what we see are different sets of values being implemented or invoked depending upon the state and the role of the person involved.

Values and norms, then, are situational rather than absolute. The nurse or the doctor who may have been quite intoxicated the night before at a party will not necessarily be tolerant of the intoxication or marijuana-smoking of a patient. The values have changed. What is acceptable behavior for the doctor or nurse in a party setting is not acceptable for the patient in a hospital setting. Any analysis of operational values on a unit, then, must take into account that values are not static but can shift radically depending upon the role and the relationship. In this instance, the shift was from external ward values (values applied outside the ward) to internal ward values (those acceptable within the ward). The same could hold true of patient values; that is, were the patients not patients but operating normally in the world, their values might well be the same as those of the doctors and nurses described. However, because they have been put into the position of being patients, their values have altered according to their new roles. On a superficial level, this may well look like hypocrisy in which we all participate, not because we choose but because we must. It would be perhaps more accurate to describe the fluctuation as a shift in perspective.

What, then, were some of the internal ward values that guided behavior on the rehabilitation unit? One of them, certainly, was autonomy or independence. There is no question that this is one of the goals for any kind of therapeutic or educational venture, at least in the United States. Observers of Russian schools (especially nursery and early grade schools) have noted that autonomy is not a universally desired trait. In contrast to the individually focused activities in

American schools, Russian schools encourage cooperative ventures and discourage competitive ones. In the United States, however, we believe that autonomy, being able to take care of oneself, is the ultimate good. We have many expressions of this value: survival training, living in the wilderness, Outward Bound, doing one's own thing. In fact, it is questionable whether one dare encourage any venture that develops dependency. Perhaps the most obvious example of our judgment against dependency comes with our attitude about children who cannot do things for themselves—they have been spoiled.

Often, however, the obsession with independence is a cover-up for indifference. A parent, for instance, may say that he wants his child to be autonomous when what he really wants is to have the child leave him alone. The wealthy or prosperous often denounce welfare on the grounds that it breeds dependency when what they are really objecting to is the use of their money for another's benefit. Similarly, on the rehabilitation ward, while autonomy was definitely a commendable value because patients were being prepared to resume their worldly lives, the value often was invoked by those who simply did not want the trouble of helping the patient. The staff were able to say that they did not need to bother with a particular patient because he was learning to be independent. It was an excuse not to have to give constant attention to a patient, and the staff could justify reduced contact and care of the patient; they could relieve themselves of certain kinds of unpleasant duties, tasks, activities, or relationships by invoking the value of independence. The result of this rationalized neglect could be seen toward the end of the unit's life, in the amount of inactivity on the ward. Patients often were seen either propped up in their wheelchairs in the corridor, or sitting in their rooms reading, or just staring vacantly into space. A great deal of neglect can be justified by invoking the prime value of independence, and with this value perhaps more than any other, a careful watch must be kept to make sure that it remains a value and does not become a demerit.

A second value intertwined with the theme of physical rehabilitation (and some psychiatric rehabilitation, as well) comes with the idea that something must hurt before it can get better. To some extent this is true in physical rehabilitation. One has to work a body part that hurts in order to get it to heal better; and while it is being worked, it might well hurt more. This value is based on a sound physical principle, though we must keep in mind that the body part is worked to the point of pain, not suffering. When a patient is made to suffer under the principle that something must hurt to get better, then we can assume that the value has been placed in the hands of a sadistic therapist.

Other internal ward values included the following: (1) it is good to help people improve; (2) it is good to work for improvement; (3) struggle and hard work are essential for improvement (a Protestant-ethic notion of hard work); (4) patients should conform to staff rules and behavioral expectations; and (5) physical rehabilitation is more important than psychosocial rehabilitation.

One conflict that occurred on the rehabilitation ward, and that probably will occur on every unit that leaves the question open, arose because of disagreement about the emphasis of the value system. Was the unit's value system to be patient-oriented or staff-oriented? Ostensibly, of course, the ward's value system was patient-oriented, though in reality it wavered. We feel that at the outset, at the opening of any medical unit, it must be made clear that we do not have a staff-oriented value system. There is no democracy within a medical unit; democracy exists outside, but it does not exist on the ward. This is not the staff's place; it is the patient's place. Staff should not be allowed to vote on what they do; this is their job and they get paid for it. The patient is the consumer, not the staff member. To place staff satisfaction higher than patient care would be to turn the whole tradition of medicine upside down.

A major source of value conflicts among staff members and patients came as a result of the wide disparity in ages both of staff (who ranged in age from the twenties to the sixties) and of patients (who ranged from fourteen to eighty years). Even in the most rigid of societies, different age groups will have different ideas about what behavior is permissible and what prohibited, what kinds of things are worth working for and how much work one should do. Obviously, then, in the relaxed atmosphere of a rehabilitation unit, these conflicts will emerge and can, if they are not controlled, become highly disruptive of the unit's routine [31].

Just as the ward imposes internal values on patients, patients impose external values on the ward [32]. Their values will affect their self-images [33, 34, 35], their attitudes toward their disorders or the hospital in general [36, 37], and their relationship with and attitudes toward the staff members [38, 39].

The younger generation on the rehabilitation unit agitated for more freedom and for fewer restrictions in dress, in allowable ways of demonstrating affection, and in the use of mind-altering drugs such as alcohol or marijuana on the ward. The older generation, on the other hand, perhaps in reaction to the youth, wanted even greater prohibition of precisely those things the younger people desired. Similarly, relationships between people are also perceived and valued differently by the older and younger generation. The younger people on the ward were more egalitarian, with much less emphasis on respect for authority; in fact, there was often a strong antipathy toward authority. They tended to be more informal; it was first-name-basis generation. The older people on the ward often were shocked by the lack of respect for accomplishments, status, and position the younger generation demonstrated.

In the main, however, the ward was founded on the values of the older generation because both the ward director and the head nurse were members of the more conservative class on the unit. Contrarily, the values of the service staff tended to be more in agreement with those of the younger generation, and this gap, as will be illustrated later, greatly affected the harmony on the unit among both staff and patients.

We discussed in Chapter 2 how the values of the hospital, the rehabilitation unit's micro-environment, affected and conflicted with the values of the unit itself, but yet another sort of environment brought value pressures to bear on the rehabilitation unit, and that environment was society at large. The hospital and the rehabilitation unit were particularly vulnerable to the values of the times—they had a door to the outside that was open to anyone who wanted to walk in from the street. And the values of those times were particularly disturbing.

This unit was in operation during the late 1960s and early 1970s, a period of great disruption in American society. These were the years of the Vietnam war, Cambodia, hippies, demonstrations on the streets and in the colleges. These were the years of social revolution by blacks and women and minority groups generally. Those who had believed they had no right to complain and no power to protest had learned that they could raise their voices and, by doing so, could effect changes in values, behavior, and practices. They learned that these changes would be supported by the courts. These were the years when it became evident that there was no practice too sacred to be questioned. Along with social and cultural traditions, pharmacological beliefs were also overturned. Whereas, formerly, most persons would have agreed that mind-altering drugs such as LSD or marijuana must damage the brain in some way and so must be bad for the individual, in this generation such mind-altering drugs and psychotic or parapsychotic experiences were highly valued. The hallucinatory experience was glorified in the popular literature. To expect that a small rehabilitation unit could be sheltered from values that were effectively creating havoc in an entire country might in itself be called a hallucination, and certainly the ward was not proof against the upheaval in values outside the unit. Angry conflicts among staff and patients resulted from these changing values. Lines were drawn and certain attributes, behavior patterns, and dress styles became symbolic of adherence to a given set of values; long hair, drug use, and peace buttons identified the new set of social loyalties and values, whereas short hair, respect for authority, and (at least seemingly) abstention from drugs came to represent adherence to the more traditional values that were under attack.

Along with conflicts in social values came conflicts in personal values. We all carry around with us our own set of values, things that make us like or dislike people, make us approve or disapprove of their behavior, make them attractive or repugnant to us. Probably the intense stratification occurring outside the ward magnified everyone's personal values, making them less able or less willing to qualify their likes and dislikes. Whatever the case, individual conflicts ran quite high on the ward, and we can conclude that personal values were given more weight than a strict adherence to a professional role would allow.

Culture

Despite the many differing roles, values, and rules that permeate an organization, much is shared among members on the unit and patients living there. This shared element, the part that overrides the differences among a group of people, is the culture, and the social equivalent to this is community or a sense of shared identity in spite of differences.

When looking at an organization like this rehabilitation unit, we can view its culture in different ways, considering how developed it was, how much was shared, and how great an impact it had.

For example, imagine a group of people who meet together for the first time in an isolated setting; for example, the well known group of shipwrecked persons meeting on a desert island. Imagine that each person came from a different ship that represented a different nation. We can assume, given these conditions, that on the first day there will be no culture shared by the whole group. Each person will have the culture he brought with him, rules that will guide and control him in certain ways, but the group as a whole will have no culture of its own. On day two, however, there already will be something shared, and by day 1,000 much more. There probably will have developed values, rituals, rules, notions of roles, and some stratification that the group generally accepts and believes is good. The group may not even be fully conscious that a culture is developing, but should a new person enter the group, he would clearly perceive the evolved culture and he would have to begin adapting to it.

We can also look at a culture qualitatively, examine the "what" of the culture, the organization, its function, its economics, what each person brought in, and unpredictable events such as disasters. It would depend on how long the organization had existed as an integral unit, how much change had taken place, how much turnover there had been in the organization (people coming and going will certainly affect what kind of culture will develop and how long it will take to develop).

We would not, however, be very successful in applying such measurements of culture to the rehabilitation unit, for the ward never evolved a culture of its own, nor was there ever a sense of community. People coming into the ward maintained their own culture; indeed, they often maintained it the more strongly if it was in opposition to the values of the unit.

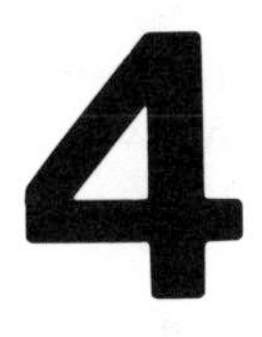

Life on the Ward

This chapter will attempt to give a sense of what life on the unit was like, what activities composed a typical day, and what sorts of interaction were common. We will look at some of the facilities the patients enjoyed and the roles families played in the unit's life, as well as at attempts that were made at structuring groups for intimacy and community among patients or between patients and staff, and groups whose purpose was to analyze problems. Finally, we will introduce a few of the patients who made the ward their home.

A Typical Day on the Rehabilitation Ward

The day on the rehabilitation ward began at about 7:30 in the morning when the night nursing staff were relieved and the day staff came on duty. The day staff were carefully briefed on the state of each patient's health, what needed to be done for him, and how he had passed the night. After the briefing, the nurses then helped the patient get ready for the day. The patient was assisted in whatever was necessary to prepare him for going into the dining room to eat breakfast. This often meant helping the patient to rise out of bed, clean himself, dress. No one who could be taken to the dining room for breakfast was allowed to stay in his room; only those who were completely bedridden were not expected to join the group. Even if a patient had to be spoon-fed, he was spoon-fed at the table with the rest of the patients. For some, generally the more healthy evaluation patients, the experience of eating with severely crippled people was at first difficult. Sometimes they felt embarrassed at being on such a unit when they were fully ambulatory and not handicapped. However, the communal eating pattern often became a growing experience for the evaluation patients, some of whom in their short stay became quite close to the regular patients, deriving pleasure from helping those who were far more debilitated than themselves.

After breakfast, everyone on the unit scattered, the nurses serving mainly as dispatchers to make sure the patients got where they were supposed to go, to the pool, to X-ray, to an electromyogram test, or to the dayroom where physical therapy continued during the entire morning and afternoon, punctuated by occasional refreshment breaks.

The patients returned to eat lunch together and then retired to their rooms for a while. Some would take naps; others would join some staff members in the dayroom, to watch soap operas on television. Then the patients would disperse again, some back to physical therapy, others to whatever was on their treatment regimen.

Daytime was not a period for social cohesion on the rehabilitation unit, the patients all being involved in carrying out the specifics of their various therapies. People entered and left the ward continuously: physicians of various specialties came to see private patients; residents and the chief of service came in to see staff patients; relatives and friends wandered in and out, visiting all afternoon (while the official visiting hours were from 2:00 to 4:00 P.M., the staff were generally liberal in allowing guests to remain beyond these hours). Some patients had visitors around a good part of the time, others almost never had visitors, and some had visitors only in the evening. Also appearing and disappearing on the ward throughout the day were the lab technicians who came to take blood, nursing supervisors to visit the nursing staff, and cleaning personnel who came to service the unit.

Some patients went out from time to time, either alone or accompanied by a relative or staff member. Those who were fully ambulatory could leave whenever they wished, as long as this did not mean neglecting their treatment. If any one word could be used to characterize a day on the rehabilitation ward, that word would be motion. Going and coming, doing this or doing that, being in one place at one time and another place at another time—from 7:30 A.M. to 4:30 P.M. this was the scene on the ward. Then, after 4:30, the ward became more quiet, movement decreased, and staff were reduced to two people.

Dinnertime marked the beginning of the end of the day; nothing else was going to happen. Patients took this meal, too, in the dining room, sometimes preparing the meals themselves in the kitchen on the ward. In general, this meal was less lively than the others, there being no expectations of future activities except evening visits from family and friends. Patients became more introspective or more talkative. Because there was time to get to know each other, the relationships between the patients and the evening staff were much closer than those with the day staff. One evening nurse allowed candles to be lighted in the patients' rooms, and she permitted the patients to have wine and marijuana (things which were in direct violation of ward rules).

By 8:30 P.M., the unit was quiet. Some patients sat watching television in the dayroom or in their private rooms, and nurses administered night medications, took care of patients' needs, or sat down to watch television themselves. By 10:00 P.M. the unit was silent. Perhaps one or two patients, usually healthier evaluation patients, still sat up watching television.

A Typical Weekend

The weekend started on Saturday morning and ended on Sunday night when those patients who were on leave returned. Most patients went home for the weekend. Because the cost of hospital care was so great, many evaluation patients entered on Monday and were gone by Friday, and those regular rehabilitation patients who were able to do so went to stay with friends and relatives. This sometimes left only one person, sometimes two or three, on the ward.

Because anyone who could leave left, to remain on the ward was both a measure of the severity of the patient's physical or emotional disability and a measure of the weakness in his social support. The weekend was a lonely and potentially depressing time for those too physically impaired to leave the unit and for those without family or friends to visit. As a result, there were many patient-staff conflicts, the staff complaining about the demands and ill humor of the patients, and the patients complaining that they were receiving no attention and no therapy.

Some effort was made to provide activities for those who remained on the unit, but the staff itself was greatly reduced. There were no physical therapists, no physicians around most of the time, though they were available if called, and the nursing staff was cut to a skeleton crew. On these days, the ward community consisted of a few patients and a few members of the nursing staff, and sometimes there was the feeling among both staff and patients that "we are the residue, the ones left behind." Even this "we" broke down, however, for the staff stayed only eight hours while the patients were there for the whole weekend.

There was a little therapeutic activity on Saturday morning but none for the remainder of the weekend. The attending physicians came for a while on Saturday mornings; then, they too left. From Saturday noon on, life was very quiet. There was a bit of excitement at mealtimes, some watching of television, and some of the staff made an effort to play games with the patients or to generate positive feelings among those left behind, but moods were not easily elevated.

Visitors were particularly important on the weekends, and both patients and staff looked forward to these interruptions of the quiet unit life. For patients, visitors represented people whom they knew and who knew them, people they loved or did not love but were in some way involved with, and people who simply changed the routine. Visitors proved to patients that they had an identity and a place outside the hospital, that those on the outside still knew and remembered them.

Equally valuable to nurses, visitors broke the monotony of the too-calm ward and they relieved the nurses for a period of time from the responsibility of having to ease the patient's sense of isolation. The presence of visitors on the ward served very much as a respite for the staff, and they were also often a source of social contact for the nurses. Frequently, relatives and nursing staff conversed and became close, so that a visitor for the patient frequently also meant a visitor for the nurse. Often the relative acted as a catalyst or lubricant for the staff's relationship with a patient, some staff members only being able to relate effectively to the patient when the relative was present.

There was a variety of visiting patterns. Some family members and friends came to the ward and visited with the patient exclusively, having little to do with others on the unit. Some visitors had little to do with the patients they ostensibly came to see but interacted almost exclusively with other patients and staff. Some families came, it seemed, mostly for themselves. They established relationships with other patients and, in a sense, used them to satisfy their own feelings of obligation. They made their visit and fulfilled their duty in coming to the hospital, but they did it with another patient, a surrogate patient, rather than the one they literally came to see. It was easier to relate to a patient with whom they were not involved emotionally and with whom they did not have a history, either pleasant or unpleasant, capable of arousing strong feeling.

Weekends effectively demonstrated who the sick people were and who the core people were who took ultimate responsibility for the patients. Only the nurses filled this role on the weekends; the doctors and the therapists were gone. The nurses became the sole source of the patients' support during these days, and the amount of support depended entirely on the personalities and dedication of the nurses themselves.

The Facilities on the Ward

A number of valuable facilities on the rehabilitation unit were not available on other units in the hospital. There was a kitchen, a hairdressing unit, a washer and dryer, and a color television set in the central dayroom. These had a distinct impact on the style and tone of life on the ward, and, in general, they served the purpose they were meant to serve—they made the ward more like a home.

Perhaps the most important facility was the kitchen, a convenience that gave those on the unit, both staff and patients, some freedom from hospital routine. It allowed them to plan and cook some of their own meals and to store food in their own refrigerator so they could get what they wanted when they wanted it. Cooking sometimes became a creative and uniting experience for staff and patients, and a good deal of fun was shared through the successes and failures of their experiments.

Food for these cooking ventures came from several sources. Sometimes the hospital kitchen supplied it in lieu of meals. Sometimes staff and patients provided it themselves (there was a small fund for this purpose). Frequently staff brought in food for the patients, and together they baked cakes or cooked a meal. Often, several people cooked dinner for everyone on the ward. This happened spontaneously rather than on a regular basis, often prompted by an informal suggestion like, "Why don't we have such and such tonight?" or "I'll bring in something tomorrow to make."

Cooking and eating relieved the monotony of the unit. It gave the patients a measure of freedom and control over their environment, made them feel that the unit was theirs; and it was a valuable source of interaction both among patients and between patients and staff. Sitting down together and eating the same food tended to bring the patients and staff closer to each other, since the latter did not generally eat on the ward.

The kitchen was also designed to be part of therapy, since the patient was being trained for independence and preparing one's own food was an important skill to relearn. An amputee, for example, would be retaught how to maneuver in a kitchen, how to perform familiar tasks in a new way. The kitchen, however, also brought problems. It ceased at some point to be a patients' place and became a refuge for the nursing staff. While its planned function was patient pleasure and therapy, the kitchen became, in effect, the nurses' place to go whenever they wanted to say or do something. That the staff could usurp the patients' place, and could do so right in front of the patients' eyes, created a good deal of dissatisfaction and anger in those who were being excluded.

The rehabilitation ward also sported a hair-washing beauty facility, and there was much staff-patient interaction involved in washing, setting, and combing-out hair. Patients were able to maintain their appearance, a positive factor in maintaining their sense of self; that is, their sense of in-the-world self as opposed to hospital self.

The washer and dryer also helped to strengthen the patients' continued sense of prior self. Patients wore street clothes, which of course had to be washed from time to time, and the patients could not just throw them into the hospital hopper and send for replacements, as was done on other units. The washer and dryer gave the patients more freedom, made the unit more like home, and again served as a therapeutic activity in that laundering one's clothes was a practical skill that would have to be regained before the patient could become autonomous.

Finally, the unit had a color television set, a unique attraction to some of the staff working in the hospital at large. The cleaning personnel, those doing the maintenance chores on both the rehabilitation unit and other units, often congregated around the television set to watch soap operas in the afternoon. From time to time, the nursing staff participated as well, though this was not generally an activity indulged in by high-status personnel.

Patients seemed far less interested than staff were in television viewing, and we need only consider the patients' condition to understand why. A patient who is not feeling well or who is depressed often finds it difficult to concentrate on a television program. For many people, television can be deadly when their spirits are low. They tend to see the various sequences separately, or they miss parts. Sometimes they look for some sign of humor or positive feeling so desperately that they try to pull more out of a program than it has to offer. The end of the program leaves them feeling cheated and let down. Thus, while there were times when the television united patients, staff, and relatives as they all sat to watch a ball game or a movie, usually it was not the patients who gathered around the television set.

Formal Staff Interactions

From one perspective, we could say that the staff met together three times every day when nurses, and frequently physical therapists, gathered to exchange information. At the least, a medical status was reported; at the most, feelings and reactions to events on the ward were shared, and incidents (such as what occurred when relatives came to visit a patient) were related. These meetings could also release built-up tension or generate enthusiasm.

Grand Rounds, however, was the major group meeting, and it was meant to include all persons who were involved with the unit. Under the direction of the ward director, this meeting took place once a week for approximately one-and-a-half hours. Initially, nearly everyone working on the unit, including the consultants, attended these meetings, though as the ward neared its end, the participation significantly declined. For the most part, the focus of these conferences was patient care.

Grand Rounds was meant to serve a number of purposes. It was to be educational, a time when residents, students, and all people working on the ward would learn something from each other; and it was also to serve as a review of the week. Patient cases were presented, either briefly or in detail, and they were discussed by the whole staff. Recommendations were then made. Sometimes new patient cases were presented, and a treatment program was designed. On occasion, a staff person would describe the case of an older patient on the ward, one who had been there for three weeks or for two or three months. The staff were then able to review and evaluate the treatment progress and to reexamine the hypotheses on which it had been based.

Grand Rounds was also meant to provide staff with an opportunity to express their own feelings, which often meant to complain. There were complaints about the way staff were used, about the inappropriateness of certain patients for the ward, about the inadequate treatment of one patient or the pampering of another, and about the lack of consulting assistance.

Finally, Grand Rounds was meant to provide an opportunity for the staff to develop a sense of the unit as a whole, to look at the map of the entire field of clinical problems.

In trying to fulfill its reasons for being, Grand Rounds ran into many problems. Frequently, some of the important functions were slighted, because the stated purpose of the meetings was to review patient care. For example, if the conference did not provide an opportunity for staff to express their feelings about a patient or his care, they became angry and felt that they had been denied the right to make contributions. If such staff needs were met, however, the majority of the meeting might be spent in discussion of a staff member's feelings toward one patient, leaving no time for discussion of the patient's treatment. Occasionally, this resulted in meetings filled with complaints and in meetings where there seemed to be no possibility of achieving closure. Frequently, one member would snap at another or become intolerant and say something hurtful. At times, people got angry at others for prolonging the discussion and diverting time from other case studies.

Important to the understanding of what actually happened in these meetings is the idea of closure. Closure is essential for some people, particularly those in the medical profession who often take a problem-oriented approach to health care. From their viewpoint, a case consists of the symptoms, the objective signs, the subjective signs, the assessment, and the program. They seek and need closure or completeness in working on their cases.

Those who have worked with groups over long periods of time, however, recognize not only that closure cannot be achieved, but that it might not even be desirable. Sometimes it is necessary to leave things hanging, to realize that human beings will continue to have problems and that, in fact, this is how it must be. Each person should be allowed to express his unhappiness or dissatisfaction without someone moving in to help him. Eric Berne [30] described this process clearly in *Games People Play*. Someone presents a problem; another presents a solution. The person who presented the problem then says, "Yes, but . . ."; the other person then presents another solution, and so it continues, ad infinitum. For people who expect to achieve closure, this can be exceedingly frustrating. Because these staff members were treating rehabilitation patients who were chronically disabled and thus peculiarly prone to the "Yes, but . . ." syndrome, staff were forced to confront it frequently.

For these reasons and others, Grand Rounds conferences frequently created rather than resolved feelings of unhappiness and dissatisfaction among the members of the staff. Because Grand Rounds was, or should have been, a vital part of the unit, an opportunity for staff to work out problems and create their own sense of community, its failure to achieve its goals left a large gap in ward morale that could not be bridged. The following notes from two Grand Rounds meetings will give the reader a sense of what the conferences were designed to achieve and some of the reasons for their failure.

Observations of the Grand Rounds meeting of November 11, 1970:

The tone of the meeting was quiet, and the discussion centered on plans for one of the patient's discharge. This patient had particularly asked for a discharge date, but the staff were unable to arrive at one. They could not decide whether the patient should be going home or to a commune, even though they had the clear feeling that the patient would not be able to tolerate life at home because of conflicts with her parents.

On rounds, this patient had requested a weekend pass to go home with her mother, and she seemed disappointed that it was granted for only one evening.

Many patients were passed over rather quickly—an amputee who was doing well, another patient with whom there was no problem, and another with a neurologic disease which gave her a chance of regaining function.

The tone of the meeting up until this time was deadly dull. The next patient talked about was Mrs. X, and the nursing staff raised the question as to what this patient, who had carcinoma with metastatic disease, was doing on the rehabilitation ward. They felt that she was getting no benefit from the ward, and that, in a sense, she was dictating her own treatment—she had insisted on being given radiotherapy. The decision made by the ward director was to discharge her to another ward, but as he stated, "I don't want to have to order anything." And, in fact, he had hoped that Mrs. X's physician would have transferred the patient on his own.

On rounds, Mrs. X had said that she had received complete relief from pain after her first radiation treatment and was ready to participate in whatever ward activities were being offered. But a conflict nevertheless arose about her ability to schedule anything because of her uncertainty about when she would be called for therapy.

The next patient discussed was Miss Y, a diabetic with a foot injury caused by an automobile accident. She refuses to let anyone touch this foot, and this has caused the physical therapist some concern. The dietician felt that she was cheating on her diet, and it was discovered that she frequently was running 4-plus sugar and occasionally some acetone in her urine. The nursing staff reported that when her parents come to visit, she runs to her bed, gets under the covers, and acts as if she were in severe pain. The question of psychiatric counseling was raised, but never engaged and never dealt with.

The consulting psychiatrist at this point arrived at the meeting.

The last patient was Mr. Z, who is a paraplegic, and his discharge date was set at about one month from today. This caused a great deal of consternation among the staff, because they felt that he was still making progress, however small, and felt that he ought to stay at least one more month. On rounds, Mr. Z had insisted that the director stop in and speak with him, and it had also been arranged that the consulting psychiatrist would evaluate Mr. Z again before his discharge became imminent.

In general, the meeting was dull, as were the rounds. The pertinent problems seemed not to have been touched on.

Observations of Grand Rounds, December 16, 1970:

The meeting was as usual devoted to the review of the patients. An air of some annoyance from the previous meeting continued, and the director made a sarcastic observation about the administrator who had visited at the last meeting. He asked the staff how they had reacted to his appearance, but no one responded.

One of the issues raised was the inability of the director or anyone else to contact the speech therapist who could be of assistance to the ward. There was considerable discussion about this, and it was decided that everyone would try to find a suitable speech therapist and that staff, nursing staff and physical therapy staff, would attempt to find some general guidelines which would be of help in dealing with an aphasic patient.

Another issue revolved around a patient who had been admitted recently and for whom a psychiatric consultation was needed. The patient sounded quite disturbed. It was clarified after the meeting that the staff had asked the consulting psychiatrist to see the patient, but he had indicated that he did not see staff patients. The issue was left hanging for about a week, and finally the referring physician decided that the liaison service should furnish a psychiatrist. To that end, a psychiatrist came to see the patient on December 15, but left no note and communicated with no one about his findings. This did not add to the reputation of the psychiatrist in staff meeting, and there was considerable bewilderment about what to do with the patient, particularly because he was a staff patient and therefore on the budget. The reaction from the director was that they should either get the patient on Medi-Cal or get him off the ward as quickly as possible, since it was felt that he might use up too much of the budget.

Another issue revolved around the admission of a patient who had been inadequately evaluated and was now on the ward. The patient was found to have a severe decubitus ulcer, had a history of a left nephrectomy, and had severe Parkinson's disease with resulting contractures in three out of the four extremities. This patient was also sporting a temperature, and it was of interest to note that the resident taking care of the patient had not even bothered to obtain a blood culture. When a blood culture was suggested, he didn't seem to realize that it was a blood culture which was being requested. A urine culture had shown a bacterial infection, and it was clear that medically this patient did not belong on the rehabilitation ward. A variety of procedures needed to be done (control of the Parkinson's disease, control of the ulcer, and a complete evaluation of the patient's urinary tract) before any rehabilitation effort could begin. Rehabilitation therapy would have been impossible for the patient in his current state.

The nursing staff clearly indicated that they wanted the patient out, and while the director seemed somewhat ambivalent about having the patient leave, he said that he would look into having the patient transferred onto another ward.

About half way through the meeting, I noticed that the specialty therapist was not in her usual corner position propped up against a pillow and discovered that she was on vacation. Later in the meeting, another woman entered and sat on the periphery. It turned out that she was the other specialty therapist and worked mostly in the physical medicine department. She had, however, seen several patients and reported on her work with three of them. The difference between her and the usual specialty therapist was profound. Points were made clearly; attention was paid to emotional aspects, physical aspects, and dexterity. She had even attempted to better a patient's relationship with his wife by taking some time to talk with the wife and explain the patient's need to use an electric shaver on his own.

It turned out that the new specialty therapist was only on the ward because the nursing staff had requested her to see several patients. They had not learned the specialty therapist was going on vacation for a week. They had received no prior notice and no provision had been made for a substitute during her absence. Needless to say, this was viewed as rather strange.

While Grand Rounds, as seen in the observations, provided a formal forum for the discussion of patient care, there was no equivalent type of conference in which staff relations was the focus. At no time was such a large-scale meeting for this purpose observed to take place. There were smaller meetings during which staff relations were discussed, specific complaints studied, and attempts made to negotiate differences, but no full-scale conference to discuss the group's relations ever occurred. As the tone of Grand Rounds indicates, a group designed to thrash out staff conflicts would have been invaluable.

The fact is, a decision had never been made about what staff relations were supposed to be. The basic assumption was that staff relations on the rehabilitation unit would resemble staff relations on general medical units, an inaccurate assumption, to say the least. Also, the culture of the medical establishment had been seriously in flux in the preceding ten years, and there was a great deal of conflict concerning the rights of various professional health-care personnel. Each group had wanted to see itself as autonomous, as having an identity of its own, and as being subordinate to no one. In such a climate, discussion of relations among different professionals could have been explosive, and staff tended to edge nervously away from such conversations, afraid that a Pandora's box would be opened and all evil would fly out into the world with only hope remaining in the bottom of the box.

Formal Patient Interactions

Several attempts were made to conduct group meetings among the patients, but none ever succeeded. A chaplaincy student tried to set up a patient group; some nurses and physical therapists tried to establish a patient community group; and one of the psychiatric consultants made a similar attempt. Among the many reasons why these efforts to form a sense of community among the patients failed, we cannot overlook the most obvious one. It is extremely difficult to create a group and have it cohere, particularly when trying to compose a whole out of such disparate parts. Most groups that succeed have at least one common element, and that element is usually either something they enjoy (a literary club, for instance) or something they feel to be of great importance (a political group). Perhaps most important, a common element is a part of each group member's chosen identity. While the rehabilitation patients did share a common ground—they were all disabled—we cannot expect that such a unifying theme would be successful unless it were combined with other unifying elements such as compatibility of age, outlook, goals, or interests. Certainly, disability was not a chosen part of these patients' identities; in fact, it was often a part they were fighting not to recognize.

Also, most people are not accustomed to working in a group. Some socially adept persons are well adapted to it, and these are the ones hostesses love to invite to their parties because they can be dropped almost anywhere, and they will be charming. But most people do not have this sort of social élan. They have a few friends, but unless they have had some experience with a group, unless they have been reassured and know exactly what the script is, they have difficulty participating. An important factor, too, is the quality of the group leader. It takes experience and talent to keep a group moving and interesting; and most of the people who attempted to lead these groups simply did not have the skills or the personality requisite for doing a good job. They either intervened too much or they lacked the techniques of an experienced leader. Additionally, the patient population was unstable, so that at times there would be seven or eight patients in a group, at other times only two, and the group members were constantly changing, as some patients were discharged and others admitted. This constitutes an exceedingly difficult, though not impossible, set of problems to be worked out before a patient group can be successful.

The Patients' Support System

The network of support from the outside varied greatly among the patients. More or less helpless, the patient depended heavily on family, friends, and in some cases social-ethnic political groups to be his arms and legs, his power and influence. Any indication to the patient that his support system was behind him signified that he still had some power and influence to move things in the world. Evidence, on the other hand, that his support system was weak or neglectful often produced depression, hopelessness, and resentment in the patient. Patients on the ward often depended on their visitors to audit their care, to guarantee that they got as good and complete services as they deserved.

In general, the patients' sources of support were not used to advantage in the rehabilitation program. One complication was that the areas of and quality of support were not uniform. Some patients, for instance, were very close to their families; others had major conflicts about any interaction with their nearest relatives. It often was difficult to discern how much a patient wanted the family to be part of the support system or how helpful the family would be.

In addition to the patients' often ambivalent attitudes toward their families, the tradition in the United States has been away from using the family in treatment. In the psychiatric tradition, the family is seen as part of the psychopathological system of the patient, not as a potential source of support. The patient is seen as the victim of a disease that began in the family; the family, therefore, becomes part of the problem, not of the solution.

By and large, even if they do not see the family as the spreaders of the disease, people working in medical settings do regard them as a nuisance. Families are seen as intruders; and given the architectural structure of the modern hospital, families do get in the way. There is generally no place for them. There is no privacy, and activities often stop when they come. Hospitals have long restricted visitors in the hours they can see the patient, and only recently have pediatric and obstetrics broken from this pattern and allowed a husband to stay overnight with his wife, who is giving birth, or allowed visitors to come and go, becoming a normal part of the flow of activities.

While hospitals have perhaps been too strict and unfeeling about the rights and needs of patients and their families, at the same time we must recognize that families can cause trouble and that a balance must be maintained. Particularly in the case of rehabilitation patients where hope is so difficult to sustain, families often indulge in magical thinking about what the hospital can and should do for their disabled member. Because their whole world has changed and changed forever (with most illnesses or accidents, the crisis is temporary and life slowly returns to its accustomed state, but the changes for rehabilitation patients and their families are permanent), families often endow the hospital with magical powers. The fact is that a rehabilitation patient, by definitiion, is no longer the functional human being who might go to college or not go to college, who might get into trouble or might not get into trouble. Even viewed most optimistically, he will be limited by his disability—he will never walk again, he will always be a bed patient, or whatever.

Initially, the hospital becomes a place where the family can send the patient and therefore, gain some sort of rest from their crisis. Everything will be done, and their duties will not go beyond visiting the patient and paying. They can avoid the prospect of minute-to-minute care of the patient, and the first period of time in the hospital is often a kind of honeymoon between patient and family. All of the family's positive feelings are directed toward the patient and all the patient's positive feelings are returned to the family. We often see a temporary reconciliation of previous animosities. But then gradually the question arises: what is to be done with the patient?

There are no good solutions, only a variety of more or less bad ones; and this is where the negative feelings begin to emerge. As the fact that the patient will never be whole again becomes a reality, the family starts to become dissatisfied with what the hospital is doing for the patient. The hospital, which began as the miracle institution, now becomes the scapegoat for frustration, resentment, and fear.

We are very romantic in this society, and we like to think that relationships are all open-ended and that there are no limits to what people will give each other. This is, of course, nonsense. Not only are there limits on what people will give each other, there are very definite limits on what people *can* give each other. Besides the finite nature of the care a family can supply to the patient, having to take care of someone brings out all of one's own care needs, and it can bring out the nastiest part of people.

Thus, we can see that the family is capable of affecting the patient in opposing ways—they can provide needed reassurance that the patient is still important and loved; and they can bring to the patient resentment, hostility, and guilt if they feel that he will require more care than they are capable of providing.

Patient Profiles

We will here give a brief description of five of the patients who lived on the rehabilitation ward. Patients are human beings with histories of their own. As will be seen, they form a motley group, differing not only in their background and aspirations but also in reactions to the staff and to the unit environment.

Perhaps, as much as anything else, they are proof of the cliché that what is one man's meat inevitably will be another man's poison.

Patient Case 1: Mr. C was a forty-two-year-old, married businessman who had suffered a spinal-cord injury and was hospitalized on the rehabilitation unit following successful surgery.

In keeping with his occupational background, Mr. C tended to see the ward as an organization; he criticized and analyzed it as if it were a business concern. He felt that the leadership on the unit was not what it should be and thought that the director should be more in charge, and preferably should be younger and more forceful. Furthermore, he thought that the leader should be more businesslike and not so concerned about what happened to the patients. He wanted more supervision, more action, and less feeling on the ward.

While complaining about inefficiency and laxness on the unit, Mr. C also complained about the pressure that was put on him to spend more time than he wished in physical therapy. Neither was he happy with what he considered to be the staff's poor handling of his disability. This complaint centered around an occasion when he started having spasms in his leg. Mr. C interpreted this as a sign that his spinal cord was coming out of shock. He became very depressed, as did his wife, when this hope was tactlessly squelched by a consultant who told him he would never walk again, and who gave him a choice of several procedures to relieve spasms in his leg. Mr. C felt strongly that whatever progress he had made up to that point had been nullified; he believed that he had begun to have some feeling in his leg but as a result of the doctor's diagnosis, he no longer had it. In other words, in contrast to his rational, businesslike manner, Mr. C probably was indulging in magical thinking, and he projected his frustration into blame of a staff person.

Patients who understand the direction and nature of their treatment often try to suggest changes in it, or in the administration of the ward in general, and although this patient thought that the doctors were good, he felt they should spend more time working directly with their patients. For example, they should watch the patients walking. He worked with the therapist each day, but he stressed that the doctor should also watch the patient walk or work out on the mat twice a week. He observed that one patient had been walking with a long leg brace, and that a doctor had watched him and suggested putting on straps, which really did some good. His only complaint about the doctors was that they were simply not around enough. This patient's story demonstrates the importance of the physician as an authority figure in approving, disapproving, and prescribing treatment.

Mr. C was highly critical of the weekend services. "With all the money it is costing, $80 per day, they should have a weekend physical therapist." He did feel that the aide had been some help to him and suggested that when the census of the ward was low, the nurses could help with physical therapy.

Furthermore, he felt that when the ward was really crowded, two physical therapists were required and one steady therapist should be available and possibly on call. He did not like the rotation system for physical therapists, pointing out that he personally had had five different therapists and that their views on ambulation were so different that one therapist would say one thing, then another therapist would suggest a completely different approach. Also, he pointed out that when the ward was full, he would sometimes have to wait in line for more than an hour before the physical therapist could get to him.

Mr. C was actively involved in ward life, with both patients and staff. He was eager to be accepted by the staff and by the other patients on the ward. He basically approved of the staff and the patients and took an interest in new patients and tried to help them. Because he was mechanically inclined he actually showed the staff and the patients how they could better rig some of the artificial devices that were used to help the patients. For example, he put together an IV pole on his wheelchair. He encouraged patients, while disapproving of those who did not try to help themselves. He considered one patient a "ringy-dingy" and thought of her as having "lost some of her marbles" because she carried several buttons (peace signs, etc.) on her purse. He was outraged at anyone who did not even want to try to improve. One patient who, when he first came, had said, "I don't want anything," was finally urged to perform tasks. Mr. C had told the patient, "You've got to get well so you can get behind the bar to serve drinks." Proudly, he noted that "now he's moving out and walking with a quad cane and in one month he'll be doing really well." However, he admitted that he had not been able to motivate this patient to work with his hands. "I'd want to get everything working if it were me."

Mr. C objected to the lack of activity in the evenings, complaining that there was very little diversion except a paperback or the television. He felt the ward was small and limited recreationally and socially, especially for single people. He praised highly one night nurse who got discount tickets for everyone to see *Hair*, claiming that this was a tremendous morale booster. He also cited an instance where a patient who had been depressed for most of his stay was taken on a picnic by some of the nurses and had been quite different ever since. More of this sort of activity, he felt, should be encouraged.

Generally speaking, Mr. C felt very positive about the staff. He felt most of them were helpful. He felt the nurses were wonderful and had never seen a nurse cross with him, though he had seen them lose their patience with other persons on the ward. In the night shift he felt people were more friendly, even down to the girl who mopped the floor; he noted that the night staff spent a few minutes talking with the patients when giving out medications, and that meant a lot to him.

In fact, although he realized the need to be accepted by a world larger than the ward, he felt loved and well cared for on the ward. He noted that a patient staying on the ward tended to be shielded and could easily remain ignorant of the real problems of the world. He might never know that there was a "race problem" because all of the blacks on the ward, patients and staff alike, "couldn't have been any nicer." He could not have asked for a more harmonious relationship. As an example, he pointed out how one of the aides had taken a tape recorder home and recorded some organ music for him.

Patient Case 2: Mr. TW was another acutely injured patient, an active member of the Third World who had been the victim of a brutal beating. Intensely involved in his minority group's struggle for greater rights and the restoration of their territory, he had been, in fact, a leader of this movement.

In many ways, Mr. TW's perception of the unit and its shortcomings reflected his own ideals as a leader. Being a committed person himself, one who had endangered his life and freedom by his political activities, he saw the staff as uninvolved and was highly critical of the leader, whom he saw as being detached. He believed they gave as little as they could during the mandatory eight hours they were on the ward, comparing them with "The Fugitive," a television character who was always on the run.

Mr. TW brought his political activism and concern for people's rights to the medical scene. He felt that morning consultations should have more depth and be directed specifically to the patient involved rather than to the other staff. He also believed that patients should be present while their cases were discussed at Grand Rounds, not only to hear what was going on, but also because the patients knew more about themselves than staff did. They thus might be able to make helpful suggestions to the "pros."

Mr. TW felt alienated from the medical perspectives of the unit's doctors, objecting to the Western tradition that separates the mind from the body and noting the superior perspective of medicine men of his cultural heritage who saw the mind and body as united.

Generally speaking, Mr. TW felt isolated and depersonalized on the ward, reviling the lack of mental stimulation. He felt he had nothing in common with the other patients and bemoaned the fact that there were no books on the ward that interested him. Because of his inability to relate to patients and staff, he felt like a "caged animal" and found none of the activities, including physical therapy, interesting.

Patient Case 3: Mr. D was a middle-aged, divorced patient who came to the unit in a confused, vulnerable state after an acute injury. Prior to hospitalization he had worked as a bartender and was on the ward as a result of a weakness on his right side from a complication of surgery for trigeminal neuralgia.

Mr. D felt the staff were too hard on him. He felt they were "constantly cracking the whip, and that made it rough to take." He complained that he got cold when he tried to move his fingers, something he could not do. But at the same time he demonstrated that he could lift his arms, something he had not been able to do when he came onto the ward. He was also critical of some of the staff who insisted he do everything for himself. Because he had felt unable to perform as demanded, he had withdrawn.

Mr. D was particularly satisfied with the pain medication he received (aspirin and codeine), and though he denied it, he probably was dependent on this medication, for he took it every four to six hours. At night he was up frequently because of the pain in his shoulder and head and he felt that the night nurse was nice and very helpful. There was no wait when he buzzed, and it seemed that she wanted to help him. He found the rest of the staff to be concerned and thoughtful, as well.

Generally speaking, Mr. D was not critical of the staff, had few articulated notions of how they should behave or how the unit should be run, and at that stage had little motivation to be autonomous. Socially he had virtually no involvement with the unit.

Patient Case 4: Ms. F was a young female who was hospitalized on the rehabilitation ward after a serious injury incurred when she fell from a building under the influence of LSD. Medically, she had little potential for recovering her ability to walk.

In many ways, Ms. F was an experienced patient. Because of a respiratory illness, she had spent much of her youth in hospitals, and it was finally discovered that she had also had polio. She finished her schooling in the hospital, and after physical therapy and whirlpool bath treatments, she regained control of her motor ability but experienced some loss of sensation. It was after this that she fell from the building.

When asked how she felt about the rehabilitation ward, she responded that there was nothing that she liked, but her dislikes were numerous. Among her objections was a feeling that the staff were insensitive to the fears and worries of the patients and that they often got resistance rather than cooperation from the patients as a result. Certainly, she felt this to be true in her own case, and the animosity between her and the head nurse lent credence to the felt reality if not the truth of her accusation. She explained that she had become terrified of falling after her injury, even from a height of three inches, and insisted that the staff, and the head nurse in particular, had disregarded her fear and from day one had expected her to do things without taking into consideration the terror and helplessness she felt.

A frequent user of drugs, Ms. F was considered by many staff to be a troublemaker on the unit. She openly admitted taking drugs but denied that she took them all the time, and it amused her that often she would be accused of being stoned when she was completely sober, and other times she was thought normal when absolutely stoned. She gleefully reported that she obtained her drugs from workers in the hospital, drugs which included LSD, mescaline, marijuana, and some "speed," and that she had never had to pay a penny for any of her supplies. Interestingly enough, once she had been released from the unit, she stopped taking drugs. She felt that much of her need to be stoned came from the suffocation she felt because of the ward environment. She hated being regimented and felt keenly the distance emotionally and philosophically between her and other people on the ward.

Described by one patient as the kind of person to whom one could openly talk, Ms. F herself seemed a very frank, outspoken person. She had many objections to make about staff persons, from the psychiatrist who she claimed asked her a lot of leading questions, looked out the window, and avoided eye contact when she talked to him, to the specialty therapist who she said was a waste and never taught her anything, to one of the orderlies from whom she received unwanted sexual advances, to the social worker who, Ms. F said, would ask, how are you, but never explain what she was to do for you. On the other hand, Ms. F particularly liked the director, who she thought was genuinely interested in the patients, and she was happy with all of the physical therapists, though she thought that the rotation policy was detrimental to therapy progress.

Ms. F formed a very close relationship with one of the nurses on the ward, and when she was released from the unit, after a short stay in another hospital, went to live with this nurse and her husband. This, of course, caused a great deal of conflict among the ward staff, since professional ethics have always dictated that such close relationships between staff and patients be avoided. Ms. F, however, said that she was very happy in the nurse's home and making much more progress there than she had ever made on the ward.

Patient Case 5: Ms. RL was on the ward for five months as a consequence of injuries received from an auto accident. During her stay, there was a great deal of controversy about her: she had lived in a commune before coming on the unit, she insisted upon following a macrobiotic diet, and in general, her philosophy and life-style were in conflict with ward values.

Just being on the ward made her feel claustrophobic, tense, and, as she described it, "crazy." Used to an outdoor life, she found it very difficult to adjust to the four-walls atmosphere of the unit, and she hated the constant people-noise that filled the ward. She disliked and was perhaps threatened by the physical orientation of the rehabilitation ward, feeling that there should be less emphasis on the body alone and more emphasis on the spirit. This, we should note, was also one of the complaints of Mr. TW. She thought, in a way, that she had been hexed by the doctors who would say, "Well, you might never walk again." By telling her such a thing, Ms. RL felt that the doctors were trying to kill her faith in her ability to heal herself and that a patient who was not strong might lose his faith in his other abilities. Her version of doctors was that they were just other human beings with some technical knowledge.

A major conflict between Ms. RL and the staff centered around her diet. She felt that in order to become whole again, a person needed to have foods that were not processed, pure air, and clear water; and she would have nothing to do with the ward diet. The dietician and she fought for a couple of months, during which she neither got the foods she considered essential to health nor ate the foods the dietician put before her. Finally, a doctor on the ward stepped in and by listening to Ms. RL's beliefs rather than automatically condemning them and by suggesting certain vegetables she might eat, he persuaded her to follow a diet that would both satisfy her philosophical beliefs and keep her well nourished. Because of this doctor's tactful intervention, Ms. RL did eventually eat fish and other foods she would not have touched when she first joined the ward.

Like Ms. F, Ms. RL had a particularly difficult time getting along with the head nurse, whose traditional authority-figure stance was repugnant to the patient. She felt that she worked better when there was no pressure on her, and that the issue of who was going to control her became a dominant theme on the ward. A believer in an unstructured life, Ms. RL felt that if someone told her to do something, she naturally had the right to ask "why?" The many ramifications of such an attitude on a hospital unit are easily imagined.

Idealistic and changeable, Ms. RL said that her goals for the future ranged from going back to school, to returning to the commune, to becoming a dancer. And while there were a few staff members to whom she became attached, Ms. RL's overall experience on the ward was negative. As she stated, "It brought out all of my nastiness."

In these cases, it is clear that the patients brought who they were outside of the unit with them onto the ward. This presented a tremendous challenge to the staff, who attempted to standardize behavior on the ward. They needed to find ways of overcoming the numerous differences among patients and of providing a sense of unity; they needed to be flexible in what they demanded from and gave to each patient; and they needed to realize that there was no one approach that would please everyone. Unfortunately, as we have already heard and as we will describe in the next chapter, the staff was not successful in meeting this challenge.

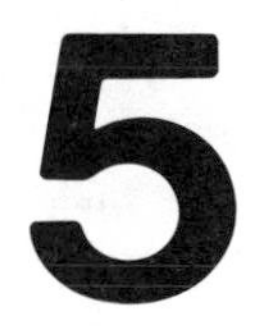

Rehabilitation Patient Roles and Rehabilitation Patient-Staff Interaction

The Patient Role

The patient is the core person in the rehabilitation unit around which all other roles presumably must revolve. The patient role can be defined as the "sick role," which Talcott Parsons [40] has described as consisting of two rights and two obligations. First, the sick person is exempted from responsibility for his illness and, second, he is exempted from full participation in his regular roles. The sick person is, in turn, obligated to consider his state of illness an undesirable one, and he is expected to seek out and cooperate with professional help.

Since any member of society can become a patient, patient groups are unusually heterogeneous, representing various sociocultural backgrounds, socioeconomic classes, and ethnic groups. As seen in the case histories presented, these patient populations bring with them a multiplicity of attitudes toward hospitals, treatment, and physicians and staff. When additional differentiating factors are introduced—such as the nature of the disease, prognosis, level of pain experienced, ability to afford treatment, preexisting relationships with physicians, and strength of family ties—we can predict that each person will react differently on a rehabilitation unit [41, 42]. What patients have in common is that they are hospitalized and that they want treatment, encouragement, and concern.

The role of the patient varies according to the type of hospital care he requires. Certain kinds of medical care demand a greater deviation from the patient's normal social role, personality, or position than do others. This can be clearly seen by comparing the patient role on a rehabilitation unit (or a psychiatric unit, which is similar) with the patient role on a medical or surgical unit. Patients on the latter wards tend to behave in a manner consistent with their usual personalities; for instance, if they have a high status outside of the hospital they will generally behave within the hospital in a manner to reflect this position. Although they will be polite and friendly to the nursing staff and physicians, they will neither be obsequious nor will they feel that they have lost any of their rights by becoming a patient. They may even continue to transact business unless medical complications forbid them to do so. These patients are in the hospital for a specific purpose. Their primary relationships are to their physicians; they are only secondarily related to the nursing staff. Most often they have no relationship to the other patients on the unit because the turnover is rapid and there is no attempt on anyone's part to create a group feeling.

The patient on the rehabilitation or psychiatric unit, however, is in a different position. Anticipating much longer stays, the staff tries to plan a social system enabling the patient to establish relationships that support him and through which he supports others. The staff tries to establish a "we are all in this together," one big family atmosphere in which the patient is expected to join. As, in a sense, he is the child in the family, the patient is expected to obey those rules the staff deem necessary for making the "family" cohere. As we saw in the last chapter, major problems arise when the patients do not agree with the basic tenets of the staff's proposed "family."

A patient should not be expected to become a member of the unit "family" immediately; this is a process that requires time. On day one, we should expect one kind of behavior and attitude toward the environment, the staff, other patients, and himself; on day 100 we should expect quite another sort of outlook. Many of the patients on this rehabilitation ward complained that they were forced to adhere to the unit rules far too quickly, particularly in areas of self-help or in areas where their fears or emotions made immediate obedience and participation difficult. Socialization into any sort of new environment is a slow process. Entering a rehabilitation unit is much the same as entering a new community, and we can speak of the patient's socialization into the roles and way of life of the unit as one of the requirements for a unit's success.

On the first day of admission to the new unit, the patient's abilities should not be diagnosed to any great extent. We should consider the patient as disabled but not necessarily sick. In fact, the patient does not know upon entry exactly what the extent or duration of his injuries is. One of the first stages, then, that a patient goes through is a period of evaluation by the staff—the medical and nursing staff and the physical and specialty therapists. The staff's position could be described as follows: "We do not yet know the extent of the patient's illness, but we are looking and trying to determine how much the healthy or functioning parts of the body can assume the abilities usually performed by the sick or disabled portions. At this moment, however, we do not have to make any decisions."

At this stage in the treatment process, patients should also be expected to be skeptical. They should be permitted to be obstreperous and to have reservations about the effectiveness of the treatment or the appropriateness of their placement on the unit. Inasmuch as the shock of first entry is often great, patients must be permitted to complain that they were not informed about certain things, that their symptoms are being ignored, or that they are not receiving the attention that they deserve. They often will want to relate their experiences prior to coming to the ward, and at this point in the therapy program, patients must be allowed to express their depression and hopelessness.

Difficult as it may be to handle an incoming patient, it must be remembered that during the initial hours of his stay on the ward, he probably is experiencing an identity crisis [43]. He has not yet perceived himself as debilitated, and one of the most difficult problems with physically disabled patients is that they view themselves as normal [44]. When they first enter the ward, they frequently look around at the other disabled persons without identifying with them. This is similar to a psychiatric unit, where patients also begin their stay by viewing the other patients on the ward as different from themselves. A mind trying to sustain its sense of a past image, a patient initially will consider himself to be more like the staff than like the other patients. However, at least for rehabilitation patients, this beginning viewpoint changes quickly, for their disability is physical and therefore apparent to all. After a short time they are no longer able to say, "We are normal," as psychiatric patients might be able to say. They and everyone else can see where the differences lie [45], and as some of the patients cannot exist by themselves for even twenty-four hours, as they are unable to move far enough to maintain essential bodily functions, their perceptions of themselves as patients are quickly achieved.

The next phase in the patient's socialization into the ward life is the learning stage. Patients become aware of the routine on the ward and begin to understand what is going to happen to them and what will be expected of them. They learn what their own daily routine will be—when they will have to get up, when the meal wagon will come around, when they will go to physical therapy, and basically what the staff will and will not do for them.

Patients often arrive on the ward with the hope that the staff are there to serve them alone. They soon discover, however, that the staff are there for other reasons and that only a small portion of staff time is actually devoted to patients. Patients also learn that staff members must share their time among many patients and that they devote some of the time to themselves as well. This often makes the patient feel disillusioned, angry, and fearful: disillusioned because he expected better, angry because he feels he is being cheated, and afraid because he becomes worried that he will not be maximally helped.

As the patients begin to develop more personal relationships with the staff and gain understanding of the ward routine, staff can then begin to expect them to cooperate with the program of physical therapy and to begin to do certain things for themselves. Although patients must acknowledge that they have some deficit or impairment, discomfort, and continuing depression and despondency, they are now also expected to display a modicum of hope. This "hope element" is essential, for it is what will motivate the patient to cooperate with the therapeutic program. A fine balance must be maintained, however, for if hope soars too high, it can be followed by an equally plummeting depression that may well undo all the progress that had been made.

Achieving the ideal sick role, then, is very much a matter of balance—balancing optimism against depression, hope against despair. The patient is expected to start at the negative end of the scale—skeptical, depressed, and often in despair—and is expected to work his way toward the positive end, where he has faith in himself and in the staff's abilities to rehabilitate him and is therefore willing to cooperate with them in the treatment program. The ideal patient will be able to move from denying and resisting to accepting and appreciating the help he is given.

The psychiatrist should be called to see the patient who does not fit into the ideal sick role—the patient who is determined that he is magically going to sprout a limb or miraculously repair himself and who therefore does not cooperate by doing the exercises, or the patient who is so depressed that he does nothing, or the patient whose dependency is so great that he can take no action by himself.

Once the patient has made the initial adjustment to ward life, his responsibilities increase. He is expected to participate fully in his treatment, be motivated, be grateful for the staff's efforts, and recognize the authority of the ward personnel and comply with their directives. These expectations are related to the patient's main reason for being on the ward—his rehabilitation. Other expectations or limitations on the patient's freedom that are not essential to fulfilling the treatment goals but are considered necessary for the cohesion of the group, the community, will also be imposed.

One of these, as we have already seen in the case of Ms. RL, is diet. Generally, hospitals do not allow patients to choose their own diet. Because they are associated with health and health care, hospitals feel that it is their responsibility to be certain that a patient has a nutritious, balanced diet while he is under their control. The patient may starve the day after he leaves the hospital or may have been eating all the wrong foods before he entered, but for the duration of his stay, a patient will be given the prescribed food. If, as in Ms. RL's case, the patient does not conform and eat that healthy diet, consternation results.

Dress and hair styles frequently are standardized on a hospital unit, and while the extreme of conformity, wearing a hospital uniform, was not required of patients on this rehabilitation ward, more subtle pressures to dress or wear one's hair a certain way were imposed. As mentioned before, dress and hair style become symbolic of attitudes toward the world in general. On this ward, people who wore certain hair styles or who dressed a certain way were considered to adhere to "hippie" practices. Hippie practices signified a disregard for all positive aspects of health and social conformity and a perverse adherence to the negative side of social behavior and the use of drugs. A hospital unit consciously and unconsciously looks for signs of subjugation to and agreement with the system. Uniformity of dress and grooming came to mean a willingness to conform to the patterns set down by the unit and traditional society at large. Deviance from this norm was accepted only with difficulty.

Theoretically, the patients on this rehabilitation unit had the freedom to come and go as they chose. In fact, however, several factors limited this freedom. Besides the obvious restraints placed on a patient's movement by his own reduced physical or mental capacity, the requirements of his therapy also restricted his freedom to move. A patient could not go off on an excursion during his treatment hours. There were few places for the patient to go, particularly if, as was often the case, the patient had limited funds and few family or friends in the area. He could go to a nearby park, or take the bus downtown, but if the patient knew no one and was unfamiliar with the environment, the pleasure of such an adventure would be greatly reduced.

A final and more controversial restriction on the patient's freedom of movement came because the staff had to approve the persons with whom the patient was going out. Generally speaking, the staff were legally exempt if they allowed the patient to go out with a seemingly responsible relative and something happened. If, however, they let the patient go out with friends, especially those they thought to be irresponsible, they were not exempt and were subject to criticism or suit. The question, of course, now arises: Upon what was such a value judgment based? Staff tended to regard as unsuitable or irresponsible those friends of a patient who, in staff's eyes, might lead the patient either to drink or to drugs, or who might not be able to take care of the patient or be fully capable of dealing with him. Responsibility on this ward, as in society in general, was equated with straightness. Even though some of the "unstraight" or "hippie" friends were the most constant and tolerant of the patients' social resources and no incidents were ever observed in which they acted irresponsibly toward a patient or endangered the patient's welfare, nevertheless, "hippie" friends were regarded with much suspicion and disapproval by many of the staff.

Patient Types

Patients are not a homogeneous group with a characteristic set of needs. Both patients and needs vary tremendously within the unit community. We can, however, for general definition purposes, group patients into types, and the first distinction we should make is between long-term rehabilitation patients and short-term or temporary patients. Within the first group, we can further distinguish three different types of long-term rehabilitation patient: (1) the acutely injured patient, alert mental state; (2) the acutely injured patient, confused mental state; and (3) the chronic, experienced patient.

Many of the patients who came to the rehabilitation unit were victims of an acute trauma or injury that had resulted in seriously disturbed anatomy and physiology. For a number of these patients, this was their first long-term experience with rehabilitation, and as they were still mentally alert, they often were very aware and sometimes highly dissatisfied with the life they found on the unit. They tended to have strong ideas about how the ward should be operated, and occasionally they had confrontations with the staff over these ideas. Mr. C., patient case 1, could be considered to fall into this category. While he was not one of the ward's prime critics, he was very vocal about the changes he felt should be made in ward policy and practice.

Unlike the mentally alert patients, who had quite clear ideas about what they liked and did not like on the unit, were those patients who perceived the ward environment and their relation to it in a confused, vague manner. These patients tended to want more than anything else stability in the environment and in their care. Because they had difficulty absorbing all the different information presented to them or integrating that information into their lives, they were grateful for the mere relief of discomfort and for simple communications from the staff, communications that did not require a complicated response. The confused patient generally accepted the kind of treatment provided without questioning whether it would build a dependency, as with drug administration, or be harmful to eventual recovery. An example of this type of patient would be Mr. D.

Chronic, experienced patients were those who had been hospitalized previously in other rehabilitation facilities. Their condition usually had stabilized and they were taking little medication. They usually had been disabled for some time and were seeking support or an additional increment of recovery. Ms. F would be considered a borderline example of a chronic, experienced patient, for while she had not been previously hospitalized for her current injuries, she had spent a great deal of time in hospitals, and had received rehabilitation treatment after her battle with polio.

In speaking with chronic, experienced patients, it became clear that their approach to the unit was different from that of patients who had never been in a rehabilitation environment. They dealt with physicians and nursing staff in much the same way as an experienced purchaser of services would bargain with his supplier. They often challenged the ward staff and wanted to be convinced of the competence of those who treated them. They refused to accept the expertise or authority of physicians and nurses as a guarantee that they would receive quality care, and soon after they arrived on the ward, they usually wanted to know if the staff were aware of their condition and previous treatment.

Chronic, experienced patients frequently took a much more active role in their health care than did other patients. They insisted upon accurate information about their condition, even though they might fear such knowledge. They tended to be acutely interested in the history and progress of their disorders, and they wanted a definite indication of what could be done to increase their functioning. Furthermore, these patients often took a highly critical approach toward their treatment and wanted to learn about and personally assess the advantages and disadvantages of any proposed therapy.

Because of their previous experience in hospitals, chronic, experienced patients also tended to develop a different sort of relationship to staff. They usually did not become as dependent on the medical staff, but instead used the staff to achieve the patient's own goals. It appears from interviews that many came to see physicians, nursing staff, and physical therapists as persons who lived in another world, the world of the well, the world of the intact. Because the patients had already accepted themselves as different, as terribly needy and dependent on others to help them execute movements, and because they already knew that for them even the simplest project would have to be subdivided into many steps, each requiring assistance, these patients had come to see other human beings much as instruments the patients needed to use.

While this attitude sometimes caused resentment from staff and other patients, we must remember that these patients were well aware of their limits and had already assessed what they would need from others. They were not, however, indifferent to the staff's good opinion and, like all patients, they wanted to be loved by those who treated them. They wanted to receive encouragement and as positive a promise as the staff could make that they would improve. They wanted to be given a clear explanation of their role on the unit and their part in the recovery mission, and they wanted to be integrated with the patient group though at the same time placed apart because of their greater experience and knowledge.

Chronic, experienced patients also tended to be active in their relationships with people outside the hospital. More practical in their outlook than other patients, they directed their energies toward mobilizing support from families and agencies. They wanted to know whether society would provide them with the care they needed. By the same token, they also wanted to receive assurance from their outside environment that they still belonged, that they had not been abandoned, and that their position in the world had not been eliminated.

The last group of patients on the rehabilitation unit were the short-term or temporary patients, those who came for evaluation. These ranged from the seriously ill to those who were able to adjust to their disabilities. Usually, short-term patients brought with them a different set of perspectives, and they did not want to be identified with the other patients on the ward. They tended to fear those patients who were more disabled than themselves, and they feared contamination from others on the unit. Indulging a species of magical thinking (superstition), they often feared that continued approximation to severely disabled patients would make them more disabled also or would make others regard them as more disabled than they wished to regard themselves. Their attitude was defensive, and these patients frequently believed that the staff would do nothing except render an opinion that might be harmful to their welfare.

Patient-Staff Interaction

The interactions and relationships that did or did not develop between patients and staff often were determined by the time of day or night the staff member worked on the ward. As has been noted, daytime nurses and staff members did not achieve the closeness to patients that was possible for those on the evening shift. Simply because of the amount of work which had to be done during the day, relationships between staff and patients tended to be casual rather than intimate. The evening staff, however, had greater opportunity to get to know the patients because the ward was quieter and there was less administrative work to be done. In this regard, the head nurse praised the evening staff:

> They (the evening staff) really did a tremendous amount of teaching and general socializing with the patients and made them feel like human beings, though they (the staff) were constantly being floated to other units because the evening supervisor felt that if you weren't constantly running around emptying bedpans and doing tasks, then you weren't working. People with disabilities need to talk, and they usually pick one person whom they can relate to better than others. Often they pick the people in the evening because there are fewer people around then. The patients aren't going to be interrupted when they're talking, and they just relate to the evening staff more as people than as staff. Most of the patients had a rather difficult time relating to me this way because of my being an authority figure there.

Night-time staff, on the other had, had almost no relationship with patients (this was also true on the psychiatric unit), and the relationships that were formed tended to consist of a few gentle (or harsh) words to the patient before he went to sleep or the attention (or lack of) he received if he was up during the night because of pain or discomfort. Mr. D, who was often up during the night because of pain, thought the night shift was generally very kind and helpful. They would come quickly when he rang for assistance and would often sit and talk to him until he could fall asleep again. For the most part, however, the night staff had little contact with the patients and tended to form relationships mostly with each other. Because attendance at daytime rounds would mean that they would lose sleep, the night shift were also removed from the day staff and the activities of the ward in general.

The position of the staff member (whether he assumed a leadership or service role) was another determinant in the sort of relationship that developed between staff and patient.

The ward director was recognized as a person of great ability with patients in general and rehabilitation patients in particular, but some of the qualities that made him so good with patients made him less effective as a leader. He had great respect for his patients and gave them a maximum amount of care and attention. In fact, quality patient care was his highest value and the main criterion by which he judged his own work and that of other personnel. Even those patients who disapproved of most of the staff, and who themselves were disapproved of no less strongly by the staff, thought that the ward director was "a groovy guy" and very sensitive to their needs.

The head nurse, however, whose previous experience had been on a regular medical unit rather than a rehabilitation unit, was not so well equipped to deal with the patients. Used to rapid turnover of patients and a task-orientation to patient care, she found the many differences in patient population, treatment, and patient-staff relationships on the rehabilitation ward difficult to adjust to, and, in many ways, she continued to see the unit's goals in much the same light as she had formerly conceived of the acute care unit's goals. She saw, for instance, the patient's independence, not the patient's care or interest, as the primary goal of the unit. This insistence on autonomy often led her into conflicts with patients. From her point of view, working for a patient's independence was her biggest job.

There were difficulties because often the patient couldn't see that you were helping him. Tempers flared. They got angry because you were insisting that they learn how to do things for themselves, and it was so difficult. They got so frustrated that it was often hard not to take it personally when they started screaming at you. In a small staff, you were always in a vulnerable place. Always.

However, others felt that the head nurse carried the independence goal to an extreme and that she actually resented dependency on the part of a patient. If a patient wanted a pillow fluffed, the head nurse would summarily tell the patient that since it was part of his treatment, he would have to do it himself. If a patient dropped something, she would merely say, "You have to learn to pick things up. When you go home, no one's going to do it for you." There seems to be a fine line between a healthy orientation toward independence as a desired goal and insistence on autonomy as a cover for disinterest or disinclination or perhaps dislike of a particular patient. The difference between the two is not an easy distinction to make.

The head nurse herself admitted that having come from acute care, sickness had a special meaning to her that often conflicted with the state of rehabilitation patients and that she had a hard time adjusting to the difference. As she described it, "You're in there practically behind closed doors, and they're not sick. The patients are not sick, they're disabled. So you tend to forget that they are patients sometimes." She noted that truly ill patients could not be taken on the unit. As quoted earlier, the head nurse also felt that patients had a harder time relating to her because she was an authority figure.

Many of the patients did indeed have a hard time relating to the head nurse. Particularly in the case of younger patients, the clashes were sometimes severe and there were continuing wars on the ward. For example, Ms. F related an incident that pointedly shows the hostility that sometimes existed. Ms. F had fallen asleep in the dayroom and awoke to find that the head nurse had placed her on the tilt machine while asleep and was throwing balls against her shoulder. This was one of Ms. F's physical-therapy exercises. Ms. F was so angry that she had been treated in this way that she refused to cooperate so long as the head nurse was throwing the balls, and so rather than go where they were supposed to go, the balls went all over the room and the head nurse had to chase after them until she was discouraged. As soon as the physical therapist took over, Ms. F began to cooperate, making her attitude toward the head nurse obvious to everyone.

The relationships between patients and staff in service roles also had their particular qualities. The service staff seemed to exercise a greater degree of influence over the patients than did other staff members, and because they were untrained in medical practice (they were all members of lower socioeconomic groups and were poorly educated) they often tended to act out their own psychological problems with the patients. The aides spent the most time with the patients, and there were thus fewer relief mechanisms available to them. They were in the position of the parent who spends all of his time with the children and cannot get away. The unprofessionalized person is likely to hope that his personal needs will be fulfilled by the patient, and when those personal needs are not fulfilled, anger, with consequent game-playing and acting-out behavior, can result.

This is particularly a problem in light of the tremendous power difference between rehabilitation patients and staff. Many of the patients were physically helpless and dependent on their caregivers; they were at the caregivers' mercy, and sometimes they were subjected to sadistic and manipulative measures. For example, Ms. F reported some game-playing by one of the orderlies on the evening shift. She did not like this man and thought he was sadistic. One evening, she called him over and asked him for a cigarette. He was smoking one at the time and brought it toward her with the lit end near her face. Holding her arms down, the orderly brought the cigarette to within a quarter inch from her lips without actually burning her. Ms. F understandably felt frightened and helpless. She also stated that, on occasions, this orderly would hold her arms down and blow into her ear, supposedly to try to excite her; he would then claim that he was only joking.

Ms. RL also had problems with this same orderly. In her words: "He sees you as a sexual object and makes many references to sex." She also saw the orderly as trying to control her, and she finally refused to participate in range-of-motion exercises with him any longer when on one occasion he gave her a weight to hold up and when she asked him to take the weight away, he would not take it until she had repeatedly begged him to do so.

One of the male patients also reported being hurt by an aide because she constantly made references to his sexual deficiencies. He called her sadistic and brutal, and felt that there should be some way of assuring the patient protection from such abuse.

From the service staff's perspective, working with rehabilitation patients was far from easy. One aide explained how, by the very nature of his role, the patient became dependent on him:

It was harder because you were doing most everything for the patient from the beginning. The personality of the patient would change and you would have an idea of the outcome whereas he would not. So, you would have to be very patient and wait for this person to reach the point you knew he would reach. It was hard because if you had eight patients, you would have to arrange your emotions toward four of them each day. If you had to lift them, you were taking the chance on messing up your own back. If they sat on a chair, you had to lift them into bed; if they were to be given exercise, you had to lift them into the tub. You had to do all this for them until they were able to do it themselves, and this was hard.

Because of the intimate nature of the contact between service staff and patients, the relationships between them were far closer to those found in a family than other relationships on the ward. The service staff helped, were burdened by, became irritated with, and often found joy in their relations with the patients. Sometimes, they also found an outlet for their own frustrations and hostilities.

Personal Relationships between Staff and Patients

On any unit—acute or chronic—patients and staff often develop personal relationships of greater intensity and affection than are professionally required. On short-term units, while such relationships are formed frequently, the patient is soon discharged and no one knows if a more prolonged relationship between staff member and patient developed. Their activities are soon outside the view of the rest of the staff and the other patients.

This is not so on rehabilitation (or psychiatric) units where patients remain for a longer time and where many close relationships are formed that cannot be hidden from other staff and patients. On the rehabilitation ward, for example, Ms. F talked about how hard it was not to form patient-doctor or patient-nurse attachments even though the relationships were supposed to remain distant. “You can’t just talk about whether it’s cloudy or sunny all the time.” Close relationships, however, sometimes shook the system and required that the leaders step in.

Some of the friendships that developed meant a great deal to the patients. They were in a hospital, removed from the people with whom they ordinarily interacted, and it was not surprising that they would try to establish new relationships in the hospital. One young male patient developed a warm friendship with a staff person and described how it felt to have someone on the staff with views similar to his, with whom he could share his feelings: “It was good to have somebody like him around that I could relate to. When I was walking on my crutches, he came with me and we would talk about the Black Panthers, singing, drugs, or sometimes we would sing and do stuff like that.”

Ms. F said she was visited by this same orderly three times when she was transferred to another hospital, and described how good this made her feel. Both of these young patients identified with the lower-ranking, less-authoritarian staff, and established closer relationships with them than with most of the other staff.

As we saw in her case history, Ms. F also formed a very close attachment to one of the nurses on the ward, a relationship that continued after the patient was discharged. Ms. F related how one of the nurses (a night nurse) was friendly to her, brought her a book, and gave her time to read. "She wasn't overly strict," Ms. F remembered, "and she allowed the patients to exercise when they felt like doing so." When Ms. F was transferred to another hospital, this nurse and her husband came to visit her. Ms. F said, "The nurse knew I couldn't stay in a hospital like that one and that I really needed to be taken care of but had no place to go." Suddenly, Ms. F said, while the nurse's husband was talking to her, the nurse asked her to come live with them. They could see that the patient was not being properly cared for. "In this other hospital," Ms. F complained, "the staff gave you nothing to drink and never bothered to turn you over. They (her friends) knew I couldn't take it—the next youngest person there was fifty-two. I could just picture myself there for thirty years. It only took me twenty minutes to figure out what kind of a place it was. They called me by my last name; I couldn't stand the formality." Ms. F said that the nurse conferred with the head nurse and the patient's family, and then took her home.

Ms. F claims not only that she has been much happier at her friends' house, but that she has made much more progress in her rehabilitation. While the therapist on the ward had told her she would never be able to put a device on her right hand alone, the patient says:

> I can do my own splint now. A visiting nurse came and showed me how to put it on, and in a little time, like twenty minutes of practice, I could do it myself. She showed me how to use the wheelchair so that I didn't need the special spokes that were on it.

Ms. F insists that she does much more now, but she does it on her own time. She often stays up until midnight or later talking to the nurse, whose husband helps her and stands by while she does push-ups.

The personal relationships that develop between professionals and patients have always been a controversial issue [46]. How close should persons in these roles be permitted to get with each other? What is wrong with a physician, a psychiatrist, a psychologist, or a nurse having a social relationship with the patient? Is it wrong for a professional to engage in a sexual relationship with the patient, or to take the patient home and establish a combination of relationships; that is, parenting, love, and companionship? Should expressions of erotic affection be permitted in a hospital?

The problem is basically one of how such relationships affect treatment. If the physician or the nurse steps out of the professional role, does that person then start using the patient for his own purposes? For example, while it should be the goal of each physician and nurse to make sure that the patient gets well, there might be some reluctance on the part of the professional to foster such recovery if love will be lost as a result of regained health. We must remember that the love relationship or friendship began in the context of a healthy, therapeutic person treating a sick person. If the patient becomes well, he may no longer need or love the health-care professional. Can the caregiver, then, allow the patient to become well? We should note at this point, however, that while this is the controversy over patient-staff relationships in general, it is not quite applicable to rehabilitation patients. Generally, the same questions can be asked and the same dilemmas pondered, but with the slight difference that most rehabilitation patients will never become well again. They can maximize their abilities, but they will always need their caregiver. As in the case of Ms. F, she will probably never be able to walk again, whatever other functions she manages to regain. While the caregiver might worry about decreased love following increased ability, he would never have to worry that the patient would no longer need his care.

It is the belief that such relationships are countertherapeutic and therefore unprofessional that makes them controversial. On the one hand, some professionals believe that if they give the patient some personal love, the patient will profit by it. The patient's motivation to work for health and his enthusiasm about his prospects of achieving it will increase. Needless to say, the patient who wants this kind of personal love and who would like to be singled out by the therapist agrees. On the other hand, there are those who feel that such relationships are countertherapeutic both for the reason just discussed and for another reason tangentially related to it. It is often feared by those who disapprove of such relationships that the patient can get the upper hand with the professional and, by threatening withdrawal of affection, coerce the caregiver into relaxing his professional standards, giving the patient drugs that will not aid his recovery, allowing him to slack off on his exercises, diet, therapy regimen, or whatever. There is no answer to this controversy. Both sides have their positive points, and the question probably will continue to provoke debate as long as there are health-care professionals and patients for them to treat.

Patient-Staff Conflicts

Patients and staff, generally speaking, agree on the basic outlines of their respective role expectations. For example, all participants in a medical setting usually agree with Parson's model of the sick role outlined in the beginning of this chapter. The model itself is not a point of conflict. Over the specifics, however, there is often much disagreement [47]. Each participant interprets the model according to his own viewpoint, his individual perspective; therefore, the model will vary depending upon who applies it. To illustrate the point, we can compare Parson's model to a model of consumers and suppliers: A seller sells a product; a customer pays for it. A seller services the product; the consumer takes care of it so it will not need excessive service. Both agree on these points. Each participant, however, will emphasize a different part. For the seller, getting paid is 90 percent of the formula; for the consumer, having the product in working order is 90 percent of the formula. The emphasis makes all the difference.

In some of the examples to follow, we will see that while the patients and staff on the rehabilitation ward agreed on the general set of rules, their unanimity broke down when it came to the specifics of the rules, the details of the sick role or the staff role. They disagreed on the specifics of what was helpful, how far the staff member should be trusted, how much of a staff person's help a patient should take, and how fully a patient or staff member should be allowed to rely on his own knowledge in any given situation.

We should note that ward life, in particular, tends to force confrontation on these potential disagreements. Residential treatment, on the other hand, differs markedly from the single doctor-patient transaction that takes place in an office. If a patient visits his private doctor, the doctor may say, "I think you ought to eat a better diet. You ought to be eating more of A, B, and C; and you ought to take D, E, and F." The patient may then go home and continue to eat exactly as he had been eating prior to the appointment. Many articles have been written about patient compliance, documenting clearly that patients frequently do not follow their doctor's advice. Sometimes they deviate from the prescription because the advice is inconvenient, sometimes because it is not part of their normal habits, and sometimes because they do not believe the doctor's diagnosis. On one level, however, obedience in a private setting does not matter, because the doctor does not see that the patient is not complying with his orders. Unless the patient looks the doctor straight in the eye and says, "I think you're a damned fool," there is no confrontation. Sometimes the physician will say, "Look, if you're going to continue smoking, there's no point in our talking about your emphysema," or, "If you continue drinking, you're going to have liver problems," but verbal threats are about the only leverage that a doctor has with a private patient, and if the threats are too graphic, the patient may well take his business elsewhere.

In the residential treatment process, however, there are constant confrontations between the professional and the patient, because in these settings the medicine-giver is also the one who makes sure the medicine is taken, the food-giver also observes whether the food has been eaten and how much of it has been consumed, and the physical therapist is present while the therapy is taking place. It is in these areas that a parental supervision pattern evolves that can create both special conflicts over values and control struggles that never have to be faced in an outpatient situation.

We have alluded to Eric Berne's three ego states: the parent ego, the adult ego, and the child ego; and we have paralleled these ego states to role behavior on a rehabilitation unit. The person acting as caregiver and authority, generally the health-care professional, can be seen as acting in the parental-ego state. The patient who is dependent, therefore receiving care and taking orders, must be regarded as acting in the child-ego state. And either person when autonomous, neither controlling nor being controlled, can be considered as acting in the adult-ego state.

One of the sources of conflict between patients and staff arose because of the difficulty some people have in shifting from parent to child to adult ego and because in a hospital situtation all three of these ego states are seldom allowed free play within one person. The professionals, for instance, must maintain a parent- or adult-ego state when interacting with the patients, though they can release the child ego to a degree when they are in contact with a superior. The patients, however, are almost completely stuck in the child- or the adult-ego state, and usually the child-ego state is the one required. Add to this the trouble many people have in moving from one ego state to another; then add also the fact that a number of people find it virtually impossible to assume one or more of the ego states, and we arrive at a situation in which confrontation is almost inevitable. Take, for instance, the case of a patient who has, prior to hospitalization, always acted in a parental capacity. If he had his way on the ward, he would continue in that role, directing and controlling everything. However, there is little or no place in a hospital unit for a patient acting in a parental capacity. Somehow this person must shift gears that he has never easily shifted before in his life, and it is only reasonable to expect that the shifting will not be smoothly done.

One of the expectations staff had of patients was that they would participate fully in the therapeutic program. This often differed from the patients' expectations, not because patients did not agree that full cooperation with the therapy program was necessary, but because the staff and patients disagreed on the semantics of "full." Organized physical therapy vs. free time was one of the recurring debates on the ward. For Mr. C, the businessman, this was a particular problem. While complaining about the laxity of the unit as an organization, he also complained about the pressure placed on him to spend the majority of his time in physical therapy. He had been enrolled in school before he was injured, and he wanted time to continue studying while he was on the ward. He had also hoped that the ward would provide recreational and social activities that he was no longer able to enjoy at home, and was disappointed that these were lacking. Mr. TW also complained that physical therapy had too prominent a place in the ward's schedule and that mental and social stimuli were given no more than a token nod. Because there was no forum in which such a conflict could be discussed, patients and staff often found themselves subverting their own overall goals because of minor differences.

Patients and staff also had conflicts over what they each regarded as therapeutic for the patients. Most frequently, the disagreement was over the use of drugs, not drugs in general but which drugs and administered by whom. Staff felt that this issue should be left entirely in their hands. Many of the patients, particularly the younger ones, disagreed. One young male patient felt that smoking marijuana had been very therapeutic for him. He had been wearing a corset he was terrified of removing because he feared he would compress his fracture further if he did. The therapists tried in vain to convince him to remove the corset while doing exercises. One day, however, while he was "stoned," he took the corset off. Thereafter, he performed his exercises and continued to improve with them. Ms. F also maintained that she was able to do far better work while she was on LSD. Both patients viewed the use of drugs as therapeutic, although the medical profession could not condone the use or abuse of them (whether legally or illegally obtained) in the absence of a concomitant plan to reduce the need for them as much as possible.

One major area of conflict between patients and staff arose over the degree of autonomy expected from a patient, how much the staff should help the patient do things he might do for himself with some effort and pain. Here, the perspectives of patient and staff and of staff among themselves were widely divergent. The patient, often overwhelmed and grieving over his condition, or having never adjusted to it, felt that he deserved some special consideration, and he often insisted that things be done for him that he might really have been able to do for himself [48]. He might see this service as one of the few "payoffs," in a sense, of his condition, in much the same way that we all expect those around us to do things for us if we are ill that we would not expect them to do if we were well. These are often things we could do ourselves—we could get up to make the coffee, for instance—but we expect others to do it for us as recompense for our illness. (In a family situation where there is reciprocity, the one who is well serves the one who is ill. In a hospital situation, of course, there is no such reciprocity.) In much the same way, the patient, while he may also hope ultimately to be autonomous, frequently expects additional care, treatment, kindness, and consideration while on the rehabilitation unit because of his illness.

The staff's position, on the other hand, is oriented toward encouraging autonomy in the patients, toward helping them achieve independence and the ability to manage on their own. Mr. D felt that the staff were much too hard on him when he first was admitted to the ward. While he was not actively seeking attention, he was still taken aback when on the second day of his stay, he was told to "do it yourself" when he requested a sandwich. The message kept coming across to him that "if you want something, do it yourself," and as he literally could not do some of the things he was told he would have to do, he became angry and withdrew.

The complications inherent in this conflict are many and difficult to diagnose, but we must first of all keep in mind the reality of the patients' condition. Rehabilitation patients are sicker and more dependent, by definition, than most other patients. They are limited; there is no question that they are limited; and they are entitled to the sick role. But they are not merely sick; they are impaired, and there is a big difference between someone who has a cancer growing in him but is walking around or someone who has had a heart attack but is walking around, and someone who cannot move a limb because he is paralyzed in some way. As a group, these are dependent people, and the rehabilitation unit must act as a place where some of the patients' dependency needs are met. The value system on which we operate, however, says that while those dependency needs have to be indulged, our function is always to meet them less and less in the hope that the needs will become fewer and fewer. The problem is not to be found in this value system. Most of the patients probably would agree with its tenets. The problem enters when each worker interprets according to his own personality and feelings toward dependency what this value system means. At one extreme we will have a worker like the nurse who took Ms. F home and who thought that patients should not have to work so hard at physical therapy. She gratified dependency needs. At the other extreme we will have a worker like the head nurse who does not want to take anyone home and for whom the whole idea of dependency is repugnant. Neither will interpret the value system outlined in the way it was meant to be interpreted, and it is likely that neither of their interpretations will be especially therapeutic for the patient.

Dependency in and of itself is difficult for many people to tolerate, and this was particularly a problem for staff in the cases where normally passive-dependent persons were admitted to the ward as patients. There was an intense amount of anger directed toward these patients, who were always asking for things, always appearing to be more helpless and needful than other patients. For instance, there was a patient with rheumatoid arthritis on the ward who decided that she was too tired to get up to do anything. As a result the physical therapist became angry with her and told her that if she could not get up to do her exercises, then she could not come into the dining room to eat. As a consequence, the patient did not get much exercise; she stayed in her room and that was it. This was an example where everyone lost because the staff member could not tolerate a nonideal patient personality.

Another example in which a patient's dependency was actually furthered by staff intolerance occurred in the case of an older patient who was learning to use crutches. The head nurse noticed her and said to the other staff, "Oh, why should we hassle? She won't learn to use a crutch; she'll be back in a wheelchair and you'll be wheeling her around. She's not the type to do that for herself." The staff, of course, then lost interest in the patient. Learning anything requires such a great expenditure of energy on the part of both patient and staff that if there is not a solid promise that the patient will use what is learned, the staff becomes unwilling to make the effort.

The staff's attitude or style often communicates to the patient whether insisted-upon autonomy is punitive or is designed to help the patient in his recovery. The approach often determines the patient's response, turning a recalcitrant patient into a cooperative one or an enthusiastic patient into an unwilling participant. For example, the head nurse's manner caused much antagonism among patients and did not tend to foster a spirit of cooperation. An instance was related by one patient, however, of a nurse who knew how to get patients to do what she wanted them to do. The patient who told this story said that one night he was ready to go to bed but could not lift his legs up to get in. He asked the nurse to lift them for him, and she said, "You know, my back hurts pretty badly tonight. You'll have to help me and try to do it yourself first." The patient did not know at the time that this was a gimmick, but it was a good idea and it worked. He lifted his legs himself.

Often, the conflicts between staff and patients occurred not because of different interpretations of ward or therapeutic policy, but because the staff tried to alter the patient's life-style and basic philosophy. The staff on a unit tend to feel responsible for every aspect of the patient's activities and behavior. They feel that unless they object to or prohibit certain activities, they are, in effect, approving them and therefore can be held responsible for their consequences. As a result, the staff try to change a patient's behavior to coincide with what they feel the behavior should be.

Behind this declared sense of responsibility, however, lies a phenomenon that often appears in an authority-subject relationship; that is, some people feel enormously threatened or offended when the behavior of others is different from their own. Perhaps someone does not eat three meals a day, or he does not take vitamins, or he does not go to church, or he does go to church–any of these seemingly innocuous differences in life patterns can cause a threatened response if the person responding feels that these actions are undermining his own life-style. Any action that causes another consciously or unconsciously to question whether his own way of doing things makes sense can cause a threatened response; and, typically, when a person is threatened, he will try to correct the situation by getting the person who has threatened him to change, to conform. This phenomenon was seen to occur repeatedly on the rehabilitation ward, where the staff tried to mold the patients into their own ideal patterns of behavior. We saw this happen with Ms. RL, who was a vegetarian in a meat-eating environment, and more controversially, we saw this happen with Ms. F, who took drugs on the ward. Any time we have a closed environment where people with different value systems must interact, we run the risk, if not the certainty, that those whose power is little will be subjugated by those whose power is great. In many other instances, however, the staff's insistence that the patients cleave to certain values was less concerned with the general medical environment for the patient's treatment than it was concerned with the individual value system of the staff person.

Lack of communication about a patient's condition also created major obstacles to the smooth interaction of patients and staff. The question of how much to tell a patient and when to tell him was a highly charged issue, and we can definitely conclude from our study of this unit that dishonesty concerning a patient's condition will only create confusion and trouble. For example, one patient on the ward had a lesion in his spinal cord. He thought that feeling would return in a month because he had initially been told that it would. He lay in bed, thinking that he felt some tingling in his foot, and he took this sensation, however slight, as a sign that he was regaining his former sensitivity. For a month this man lay on the ward, becoming more and more furious with the ward director and the staff. Meanwhile, no one would tell him that he was not going to regain function, that his limitations were permanent, and that he would have to learn to accept his disability. As a result, the entire staff was immobilized, the family was immobilized, and the patient, who thought that he should be getting better by lying there, found that in fact he was getting worse. This is an instance of what can and did happen when the physician and patient do not have an honest relationship, and this is only one example of many such situations that occurred on the ward.

Similarly, patients often were told one thing by one staff member and another thing by another. Hope would be offered by one hand, and another hand would come along and take it away. Or, as in the case of one patient who came on the ward to have work done on her leg device, the ward director told her that a cast would be made and she would be able to leave the same day. The head nurse then had to retract the director's promise and inform the woman that it would be two or three days before she could leave even though she was not prepared for such a long stay.

The staff, particularly the subleaders and nursing staff, complained bitterly about this lack of open communication between physicians and patients, emphasizing the difficulty of dealing with patients who were unaware of the true state of their disability or how or to what extent they would recover. Needless to say, the patients were unhappy with the situation, feeling that they had been betrayed by those whom it was essential they trust. This is a problem pertinent not only to the rehabilitation ward but to hospitals in general, and we will here make a case for honesty in dealing with patients. If the policy is to tell the truth no matter what, the directive is clear, and staff members will know how to act. Whenever the truth is suppressed, confusion and contradiction will follow. This is true in a family when children have to lie because family feelings and actions are kept covert rather than being brought out in the open, and it is true on a hospital unit when a patient is unaware of or misinformed about his condition and, as a result, no one who works with the patient knows what he can be told or what he has been told. Since the patient will have to learn to live with his disability anyway, and since it is impossible to work with a patient who thinks reality lies in one direction when everyone else knows that it lies in another, it seems essential for the effective treatment of the patient and the smooth running of the unit that communication between patient and staff be direct and truthful.

The question of confidentiality also caused problems on the ward. While confidentiality is an acknowledged right of all patients, it is easier to respect this right in a single doctor-patient transaction than it is on a rehabilitation unit. The demands of team treatment and therefore team consultation on the one hand, and the unit's attempt to control illegal behavior on the other, often led to breaches in patient-staff confidence. Reflecting back on her experiences on the ward, Ms. F described the unit as almost like a prison: "You never knew if you told a doctor such as one of the residents something which you thought was confidential, whether he would tell everyone else or not. Usually, the next day everybody on the staff would be coming in and asking you something about it. This wasn't right." She felt the same way about a certain physician; whenever she told him something, it would be retold to other people. At one point, she claimed, a letter was sent to her parents without her knowledge, telling them that she took drugs. She was extremely annoyed at this because her parents were very conservative and there were a number of things about her life which she had kept from them. As she said, she at least would have liked the chance to prepare them for such a disclosure rather than having it happen the way that it did.

Sometimes the conflicts between patients and staff, the gaps in values and expectations, or the unhappiness resulting from communication problems were so great that no reconciliation was possible. The patient's entire stay, then, became one of trial until his discharge. In other cases, however, as patients and staff explored their differences, either together or with the assistance of an outside person, they managed to compromise on a program agreeable to both. Sometimes a "love affair" evolved between patients and staff where the staff would see the patient as the ideal rehabilitation candidate and the patient, in turn, would see the staff as ideal health professionals. They would then work vigorously together. Whether more rehabilitation progress was actually made in these cases remains unclear because in their enthusiasm for each other, patients and staff tended to see even the smallest increment of improvement as a miraculous advance.

Generally, the relationship pattern between staff and patients became relatively fixed by the end of the second week of rehabilitation, and it seemed the case throughout that those factors that made for good relationships between patients and staff were very much the same as those that would attract the same people to each other outside of the rehabilitation setting.

On the whole, most patient-staff conflicts arose because the contracts between patients and staff were neither clearly defined nor specifically defined. By an open and well-defined contract, we mean one in which both parties overtly agree without euphemism and without complaint that there are certain things staff will do for the patient because he is unable to do them at this time, and that there are certain things the patient will do for himself because he is able to do them at this time and because doing them now will increase his ability to do them better in the future. The contract will also clearly define the patient's freedoms and restraints, and the communication pattern that will be maintained between patient and staff.

Although our entire society operates on the basis of contracts, we in medicine are somewhat reluctant to enter into contracts with our patients. We seem to think that there is something cold and unfeeling about establishing contracts that have to do with time, money, or services. Instead, we prefer to make believe that we are one big happy family, we and our patients, and that of course we will do everything for each other. Whether in a family, in a marriage, or in a hospital, such contracts seem to lead only to misunderstanding, disappointment, frustration, anger, and acting out. Any time we see acting out, on the part either of staff or of patients, we should immediately reexamine the contract. It is probable that one or both parties to the contract will have read it differently and will have contradicting expectations.

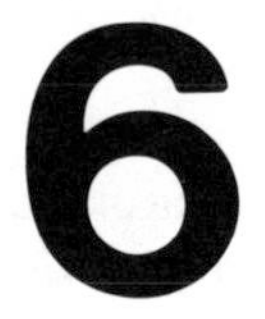

Systemic Problems That Led to the Unit's Demise

The problems and conflicts between patients and staff already described threatened the therapeutic success of the rehabilitation unit. Other problems that were systemic problems threatened its organizational survival and foreshadowed its eventual demise.

The unit was not planned or operated with any concept of the structure, function, and dynamics of an organization, so there was no view of the unit as a system. Neither were there any clear notions of the goals and objectives of the unit or how they were to be established, maintained, or revised. There was little systematic consideration of how each aspect of the unit would contribute to the ward's success or failure. Had there been more analysis, some of the difficulties, such as the problem of estimating the potential income of the unit and measuring the possibility of attaining that income, might have been anticipated. A systematic analysis could have anticipated how patients would be referred and accepted, and it would have led to standards for maintaining a constant patient population. Staffing patterns could have been examined and changes in assignments made. That there would be a need for a "board of directors" to review periodically the profits and losses of the unit, the objectives that had been met, and the expectations that were as yet unfulfilled, could also have been recognized.

The absence of a systems approach proved in many ways fatal to the unit, for one key factor in the termination of the rehabilitation ward was that even though the people concerned saw that it was not working out as planned and that it was doomed if something did not change, no one was able to bring about any changes. The system had no way to correct itself.

Census Problems

One continuing anxiety that plagued the unit came from a need to maintain full occupancy. For the director, this ultimately proved to be an insurmountable difficulty and a constant source of pressure from the administration. The establishment of any specialized unit represents a large commitment on the part of hospital administrators. Since a specialized unit in the hospital does not accept the usual medical or surgical patient, the ward census becomes dependent on one type of patient. When such patients are not referred to the unit, the census drops and the cost per patient rises. As a consequence, the administrator has immediate financial problems.

No one had ever expected that the unit would actually support itself, and the university had expected to provide support because of the ward's teaching value and utility for medical faculty and community physicians. But the ward had to be kept full. The director knew that staff support and supplies would be reduced if the ward census dropped too low. He also knew that when the census dropped, the rehabilitation ward nurses would be "floated" to other units, and this represented a potentially serious morale problem. Therefore, as we have discussed earlier, the director felt he had sometimes to admit patients who were not up to his standards or the standards of the nursing staff, creating conflicts between himself and the nurses.

According to the administrators, however, it was not the census drop that created problems between the administration and the director, but the lack of planning and control over patient population:

> The administration was concerned about the census and finances, but the real problem came because the director and the residents were constantly being called to the Utilization Review Committee to justify why they kept patients there so long. As a result, they would tell the rounds group that they were being pressured because of census. Well, that wasn't true at all. The real pressure was felt by the Utilization Committee. The director was there before the committee because he either kept the patients too long or let them come on the ward inappropriately in the first place. This committee is specifically set up to review Medicare and Medi-Cal. That's where the real pressure was coming at the director. There was no serious concern about the census problem until it became obviously futile to keep a full staff there for two patients.

In view of this administrator's statement we must consider whether there existed a real demand for the unit's services. A need clearly was present and, in retrospect, a demand probably was potentially present, also.

Demand, however, is a dynamic process. It changes from day to day. It does not simply exist or not exist, in any permanent sense. It can be fostered and developed, or it can be discouraged and allowed to decline. The demand for this rehabilitation unit needed to be fostered, and some system should have been formed to work through those problems that would discourage demand. The initial lack of conceptualizing or of anticipating that problems would arise was one of the deterrents to fostering demand. Another was that this kind of analysis is very time-consuming for the staff, and time is money. The funds necessary for a thorough systems analysis were not available, though it is clear that without such an analysis, the success of the unit was jeopardized.

It is probable also that not enough public-relations work was done to foster demand, and this might be in part because of the essential integrity and honesty of the people on the unit. For example, having been highly successful on the basis of his competence as a physician, the ward director had never had to do any significant amount of public-relations work. He had never needed to sell his product; his very integrity, honesty, and competence had produced the image of a physician people would seek out. But, of course, patients had been referred to him for consultation or treatment only—a very low-cost product. Referring a patient for inpatient, long-term residential treatment was a different matter and, as it was much more expensive, its benefits needed to be advertised.

Problems in Admission and Discharge Standards

We have already discussed the problems the director encountered in relation to patient admissions, and the complaints he received from all quarters about the patients he admitted. In a sense, he was asked to find patients who would fill beds in a perfectly distributed way to please the nursing staff, the house staff, students, the administration, and the general medical community. The director's response was a very unclear set of guidelines or standards for patient admission and discharge. The result was that the head nurse was able to assume a good deal of the control over admissions. She was known to have refused admission to certain patients, and when asked if this were not an unusual responsibility for a head nurse, she responded:

> Maybe to flat out refuse, yes, but we are not geared to taking care of acute patients. We often will tell the physician that this patient really shouldn't be here because we can't care for her, and then if we give him a satisfactory reason, he'll transfer her to wherever. Often, if it's a really acute patient, the nurse will be the one to instigate the transfer to intensive care. But to flatly refuse a patient and say, "No, I can't take her," probably is unusual.

Admitting that she did follow certain practices that helped her to control admissions, the head nurse explained:

> We would talk to potential patients about rehabilitation and tell them what to expect. Also, we sort of assessed and evaluated the situation as to whether they really were good rehabilitation candidates. The director and I had discussed it before the unit was ever opened and he said, "Yes, it is a great idea." But he never bothered to tell us before patients came.

Because her assistance in patient screening was not invited, the head nurse began to evaluate the patients on her own. She said that she felt the patients needed to know something about rehabilitation in advance, and she stated: "It gave us a chance to talk with the families, to tell them to bring clothes, and to tell them the visiting hours were different and that the philosophy was different." In fact, she was screening patients for admission. Those she felt to be inappropriate, she rejected:

One doctor in the hospital had orthopedic patients and he often insisted that we should take his back pain patients who would be on bed rest and in traction. I would say no because they're not rehabilitation patients. If there were no other beds for them, then OK, but when they could find a bed somplace else, I didn't take them, or I'd take them and try to get them moved. So you can't really say that I would refuse ever to take a patient . . . it was just the type of patient.

Because admission standards were so loose and because the head nurse was therefore able to impose her own standards of patient selection, a major eruption occurred between the head nurse and one of the residents, a dispute that, according to the hospital administrator, soured relations between them permanently. The resident had tried to admit a patient to the ward and the head nurse had refused the patient, saying that she was too acutely ill to be properly cared for on a ward that had neither oxygen nor suction facilities. From the head nurse's view:

The patient was an eighty-eight-year-old woman who had had a hip pinning. She had cardiac problems and had a respiratory arrest at the time of her surgery. She went from surgery immediately to the intensive care unit where she stayed for three days. Then she was transferred out and the physician wanted to transfer her immediately from intensive care to us. She was still on IV, she needed to be suctioned, and she needed a mist mask or oxygen continuously. I refused to take her because we had no emergency equipment. We didn't keep IV solutions there and we didn't have oxygen or suction in the rooms. She was going to be a bed patient and we didn't have the staff to care for bed patients.

When the ward would not accept the patient, the referring physician began battling with the head nurse; when he did not conquer, he went away and never referred another patient to the ward again. We must add, in the head nurse's behalf, that the rejected patient died a short while later on another ward. But, while the patient was not good rehabilitation material and perhaps could not have been properly cared for on the rehabilitation unit, still it was the director's responsibility to refuse the patient, not the head nurse's.

For the hospital administrator concerned with expenditures, the lack of clear discharge procedures was even more troubling than the laxity of the admissions procedures. He described one incident common on the rehabilitation unit:

Everyone decided that the social worker would make arrangements with the family and the director would say, "OK, next week we'll have a discharge conference." Five more days would go by at one hundred and so many dollars a day. It's likely that these were the cases that the director was called back upstairs for, because after the patient achieved all his possible potential for gain, he was still kept on.

As we can clearly see from these examples, a specific policy for admitting and discharging patients was needed, a system that could be applied, adhered to, and defended.

Problems of Staff Quality

The cliché, "a chain is only as strong as its weakest link," has many applications, one of which can be seen in the quality of staff on any medical unit. A system is needed that can both recruit people who work effectively and control those who do not, either by pulling the dysfunctional worker back into line or by dismissing him. For many reasons discussed earlier, this rehabilitation unit was not able to evolve such a system and as a result was burdened with inappropriate or poor-quality staff, a multitude of weak links.

The director could not hire or fire at will. In fact, he could not fire at all. The results of this restriction on the director's authority were evident in the example of the specialty therapist, a prototype unintegrated worker who became the scapegoat for staff and patients alike. Can a unit hope to maintain unity or preserve morale when a worker who has been deemed dysfunctional is allowed to remain on the job?

The residents on the ward were generally not of the highest quality because physical medicine and rehabilitation is one of the least sought-after areas for residency. Those assigned to the ward often were unenthusiastic and not interested in rehabilitation medicine. Can a unit hope to maintain staff involvement and dedication when the residents assigned show so little inclination or aptitude for the job?

Because the specialty of rehabilitation medicine was in its infancy, there were no trained rehabilitation nurses available. This included the role—the very important role—of the head nurse. Can a unit hope to maintain a level of expertise when there are no experts to draw upon?

The rotation of physical therapists satisfied the teaching function of the unit but had a detrimental effect on the quality of patient care and was a definite obstacle to creating any team feeling. Which, then, is to be the goal of the unit—staff satisfaction or patient satisfaction? Is there any way in which both could have been achieved more successfully?

The leader himself created many problems because of his attitude that quality work was a natural rather than a nurtured product. He hoped that each member of his staff would overcome his own deficits, would by practice or prayer or willpower learn to do those things that he could not do, want to do things he had never wanted to do before, and ultimately achieve a level that could be judged ideal. But how can one run an outstanding unit if a significant number of staff members are of inferior quality because of deficiencies in training, personality, or motivation?

Leadership Problems

The ward director came to his position with no prior experience in inpatient treatment. He did not confront the problem of dealing with or managing the human relationships on this unit because he tended to deny that there should be problems. This was reflected in the way he hired staff:

I looked for people who were more flexible in their personalities. To me that was more important than their being knowledgeable in rehabilitation. I would send them to a center to make them knowledgeable, but once they had a fixed personality, there is just no way of changing them. The head nurse was that way. She, incidentally, did not have any friction with me; she had her frictions with orthopedics. I was critical of her simply because of her attitude with other people. And I felt that we needed the cooperation of orthopedics and that she should be more flexible; but she wouldn't give in.

Unfortunately, people do not always do what they are supposed to do, even if their personalities are flexible, and if people do not expect problems, then they resent having to cope with them. Some blame themselves and become depressed; others blame someone else and become angry. Still another reaction is to see life as disorderly and unpredictable and then to become anxious. Because the ward director did not expect any problems, he became angry and anxious when they occurred, and he tended to see the problems as caused by others who were not doing what they were supposed to do. In fact, he thought that the individual staff person should cope with and rectify any conflict that occurred on the unit:

If you feel that you are interfering with the smooth operation of a department for one reason or another and there's no way you want to compromise, then you should move on to something else. I think this was obvious to the head nurse. She should have done it without even being asked; she should have asked for a transfer, but she didn't want to. I think she was as fond of that unit as I was. I can't blame her for that. She was a very competent nurse and knowledgeable in this area and she liked what she was doing on the ward. She just didn't want to give it up.

But neither did the ward director.

From his perspective, the director experienced several problems in running the unit. He felt that interference from outside authorities kept him from having sufficient control to operate the unit effectively. He explained his initial problems in setting up the ward:

For a short period of time we did not occupy all the beds, and I had the impression that this alarmed the hospital administration. They were worried that financially we would create a large deficit when the hospital had a hard time maintaining its solvency. They precipitously sought to prevent continuation of this deficit type of operation by pressuring us to take more NIC patients. The Department of Orthopedics did not wish to refer patients to us because of our head nurse; the department had had previous experience with her when she was operating on another ward, so they refused to refer patients to us as long as she was there.

He added, "I had no control over it from the beginning. From now on, I would never undertake any organization without having complete authority over it."

The director was also aware of covert actions to undermine his authority from within the ward. He was quite sure that the head nurse was disobeying his instructions regarding patient admissions. By bits and pieces, the leader was able to discover how his admission orders were being circumvented:

After examining the patient, I decided that the patient was a good candidate for rehabilitation, and I would put a note in the nurses' notes that the patient was to be referred to the ward with the approval of the primary physician. Two days would go by and the patient hadn't been transferred yet. When I investigated to find out what happened, I would find that they'd say, "Oh, the patient did not have funds to be transferred," or "The patient's relatives did not wish to have the patient transferred over here." There would be one excuse or another. But then later on I found out that really the head nurse did not want that patient on the ward. She didn't think this patient would be a good candidate for rehabilitation, and then she would talk to the social worker and to the other people and she'd prevent this patient's transfer. This happened repeatedly. I can't openly accuse her because you can't put your finger on it. All I know for sure is that something stopped the patient from going from one ward to this one and that this would happen often enough that by talking to the head nurse, she would say, "That patient wasn't good for us anyway." I might get that much out of her. I became very suspicious.

When asked how many patients were turned away as a result of the head nurse's actions, the director replied:

My guess would be two per month, and these would tend to be mostly paraplegics. Usually the head nurse objected to patients who were really disabled and whose rehabilitation potential was small in her opinion. She primarily objected to that, whereas the rest of us had a much broader attitude. On many occasions, she had been wrong. After the patient came to the ward and was exposed to the program, he showed potential that even I was not aware existed. So, I'm always willing to give it a try even though I might be pessimistic about the rehabilitation potential. Those kinds of patients she could resist.

The director, however, failed to step in and correct the situation of the head nurse's usurpation of admission power. He seemed to have little conception of how to work through organizational difficulties. He described his response to the head nurse's actions this way:

If I tried to exert my authority, I would have a disagreeable person on my hands every day of the week. I didn't want to, because she could be very disagreeable. You never knew in the mornings if she would say hello to you or not, and she was moody. I don't want that kind of situation on my hands all the time, every day, and I figured that since she was there and since I did not have the authority to hire and fire people, I would have to live with it.

Because the ward director could not bring himself to confront the head nurse and face her wrath, he probably lost a great deal in the eyes of those who worked under him. He also lost much of his already limited power.

While the director complained of his lack of autonomy because of outside interference, the outside authorities also refrained from taking over final authority. This could be seen in the case of a particular worker who many felt should be transferred. The director would not again take the case to the grievance committee. The hospital administrator described his efforts to intervene and alter the situation:

One of the first things I tackled was this personnel problem. I started this almost year-long process of giving her a list of things I wanted to see her accomplish. I said to her, "These things that need to be done are all measurable and I'm going to look at them in another ninety days, three months, after which time if you are not carrying out these things, we're going to discuss some changes which may include moving you to another unit or changing your position or whatever."

After three months, she was doing relatively few of the things I had listed. I went to the director and said, "OK, now I've reached the point where you as her superior have to get involved." I wanted him to verify from a medical supervisor's point of view that these things were not being done. He absolutely refused, wanted nothing to do with it. He had had a past history of problems of this kind and he would not get involved again.

Generally speaking, the hospital administrator was concerned with what he perceived as a lack of organizational leadership by the director. He did not really consider the director to be the kind of person who could effectively direct a unit that included twenty to thirty therapists.

The very qualities that made the director so successful with patients also may have been qualities that interfered with his effectiveness as a leader. Certainly, the satisfaction he gained from patient appreciation tended to compensate for his administrative deficiencies and consequently made it less necessary for him to correct those deficiencies. His ability with patients, the respect patients had for him, and the respect he gained from others for his treatment of patients protected him from much criticism, from pressure, and also from any feeling of responsibility for examining his leadership and his interaction with staff. He could rationalize that since he took good care of his patients, which was really the end product of the whole operation, he therefore did a good job.

In a sense, he let the leader's role slip by, because the whole unit became his patient.

However, the entire responsibility for leadership problems cannot be placed on the director himself; many of the problems arose because there was no leadership design anywhere in the hospital setting that could have been borrowed and applied to the rehabilitation unit. The design of the orthopedic service and medical services were not applicable, and the design of the psychiatry unit could not be utilized. There were simply too many leaders, and each of them had a finger in the rehabilitation pie. No single leadership model was ever agreed upon by the different leadership parties—the designated leader, the hospital administration, the medical administration, and the nursing administration. The five years during which the unit existed were filled with multiple political campaigns, pseudoelections, insurrections, and revolutions. It is no wonder that a practical model for leadership emerged and, in the absence of a specified design, it finally made little difference whether or not the leader was able to hire and fire his own staff. Inevitably, the lack of organization would have made for staff dissatisfaction and power struggles.

Value or "Culture of Care" Problems

The lack of any overriding philosophy or "culture of care" that could serve to unite this heterogeneous staff and patient population caused major difficulties on the ward. Instead of a common set of values that would unite the group, a variety of attitudes, values, and goals flourished among the staff and patients, leading to disunity and conflict. Many of the leaders and subleaders did not see any need for a clearly conceived set of values and goals for a system as small as the one in which they worked. Thus, the director did not coordinate any particular plan for the unit but saw his work as a continuation of what he had already been doing in a number of other areas in the hospital. Consequently, the staff were given a free rein to act in accordance with their own individual beliefs and priorities. Inevitably, the result was a medley of values, none with a clear lead in dictating ward policy.

A basic conflict arose because of disagreement about the value of rehabilitating certain patients. This, in turn, affected such a patient's approach to his own rehabilitation. For example, a nurse who saw little value in rehabilitating severely disabled patients might make harsh demands upon a patient to improve or withdraw from the unit. The director, on the other hand, considering that the same patient had potential for partial or complete rehabilitation, would express encouragement and optimism to the patient, who might then be motivated to cooperate and work toward self-improvement.

What was the general impact of these divergent values on patient care? Obviously, if staff members have different attitudes, the patients have no way of knowing which set of values applies to them. They might select one set over the other, but there is always a residual doubt about whether they have chosen correctly. Conflict of values among staff creates questions in the patients' minds about the expertise of those who are directing the course of their rehabilitation. Patients want a program in which they can believe, even if they do not like the demands that program imposes upon them. It is harder to believe in a program or in a solution if the experts themselves disagree.

In any organizational situation, there will be gaps between the ideal—the concepts of how things should be—and the real—the way things actually are. Overtly, for instance, the value of being friendly and supportive of each other was important. Covertly, however, that value translated itself into minor harassment and teasing. Similarly, while it was unacceptable to make a direct statement about another staff member's incompetence, staff frequently talked about colleagues behind their backs. One of the ward ideals was to use fully the time spent by each member on the ward. Much time, however, was wasted in inefficient scheduling, staff coming in late or too tired to work, and in socializing. This behavior was accepted because one of the staff's covert values was adherence to the club instinct: "We all belong to a kind of club behind these doors and we have to protect ourselves and each other by covering up for other members when necessary." "Don't take anything too seriously" was another important value on the rehabilitation unit, at least on a tacit level. Perhaps such a value originated because the seriousness and sadness of the patients' problems had to be tempered by some internally imposed attitude just to keep the staff's morale from sinking too low.

Staff on the unit filled several roles, each role type tending to have its own characteristic values. The following example shows how these differences in values were acted out on a behavioral level. It also suggests the need for specific values and rituals, a defined culture appropriate to the population on a therapeutic ward.

A Christmas party took place on the ward yearly, a party the staff were by no means united in wanting to have, but that came about anyway, for various reasons. One party was described as follows:

> The nursing staff busied themselves in setting out refreshments. The night nurse sat off by herself and said that the aide was not coming to the party for reasons she did not know. Other staffers started coming in and another night nurse brought in some friends to play the guitar.
>
> Refreshments were served and we drifted toward the dining room. The physical therapist began playing the piano and a group of people gathered around singing, including one of the patients.
>
> There was a lot of food and there were many tasty items on the menu. I felt, however, that this party was not so much for the patients as for the staff. And at the same time, I did not have the feeling that the staff was really enjoying the party. It was a disjointed experience, with some of the staff at the end of the hall where the piano was, and other people sitting and watching television.

> Later on, Santa Claus (actually the porter) distributed all the presents that people had brought for each other and also the presents that had been purchased for the patients. By this time, the director and one of the physicians had already left, although it was only 8:30. I don't recall any unifying experience at the party except when Santa Claus gave out the presents. At no time did any member of the central staff, such as the director or the head nurse, say something to the entire group of patients.

It would seem from this account that the staff's values dictated that there must be a party and that it represented a necessary symbolic chore, something that had to be done for the patients to celebrate the holiday. The leadership staff did not even seem to want to participate in the formalities of the party—the distribution of gifts, conversation with patients, or serving of food. The night nurse and the porter, staff whose values were closest to those of the younger patients, participated in the party much more wholeheartedly, encouraging the patients to share and enjoy the occasion together.

The problem with the Christmas party was that it ignored the realities of the patients' situation. It was an anomaly on the ward. The party tried to assume a "normal" stance, a pretense that "we are just like any other people who work together and have common functions; therefore we are going to have a Christmas party." The Christmas season seemed to produce a sense of guilt on the part of the staff, guilt that they were whole while the patients were not, guilt that they had homes and families and friends with whom to celebrate the holidays while the patients were left on the ward. Instead of being able to meet with the patients, recognize their plight and the staff's situation, and then perhaps decide that a party was inappropriate, the staff chose to adopt the traditional (though here ill-fitting) approach to making a statement of goodwill, the Christmas party.

An even more obvious example of the staff's application of inappropriate values to the rehabilitation ward can be seen in the description of another party, this time an Easter party. The head nurse, in effect, lined all the patients up and told them to color Easter eggs, so they all sat around and colored Easter eggs. The image of grown men and women, even if they are whole, all clustered together painting little eggs, has a touch of the ludicrous. And on this ward, some of the patients were offended at the both difficult and undignified nature of what they were asked to do. They felt, perhaps rightly, that they were being made to look ridiculous. Contrast this to the wine parties that were given initially whenever one of the physical therapists was ready to be rotated off the ward. These parties were characterized by conversation, warmth, and wine, and the patients thoroughly enjoyed them. However, these parties were soon outlawed because the nurses did not want the added trouble of dealing with possibly tipsy patients.

The conflicts and problem areas that kept any sense of culture or community from evolving on this rehabilitation ward can be summarized: lack of a well-considered physical plan for the unit, disparity in experience and competence of the workers, lack of autonomy in decision- and policymaking, loyalty division created by the temporary or part-time status for many of the staff, and the general upheaval in values that was taking place outside the ward. Add to these the peculiarly isolating nature of the patients' sickness, the vague nature of role definitions, the essential heterogeneity of the staff and patients, and the lack of well-defined contracts both among staff and between staff and patients. Add also the absence of any regularly scheduled meetings that might have released group tension and promoted team spirit, the infancy of rehabilitation medicine, and, finally, disagreement over the rehabilitation goals themselves.

This is an extensive list of problems, many of which might have been avoided by a careful systems analysis before the unit's inception and by continuing analysis during the unit's life.

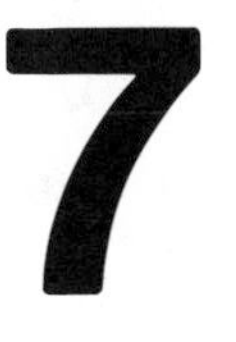

Phasing Out the Rehabilitation Unit

Despite the accumulation of worrisome problems that in fact mark the gradual beginning of the process of phasing out a unit such as the rehabilitation unit, its actual demise may occur so suddenly as to surprise those responsible for its management.

The Phasing-Out Process

Many people regard a medical unit, or any system for that matter, as an organism, as a live, indivisible whole. This is a fiction, of a sort, but it is true as long as people think it true. When they cease to believe in the essential wholeness of a system, or when a unit begins to fall apart, several things happen, many of them on a tacit and perhaps unconscious level. This was observed on the rehabilitation unit. There was a kind of nervousness among the members of the unit that if the unit died, they might be dragged down with it. There was a sense of being marked as part of a dying entity, the stigma of being a loser. There was also an irrational though very human sense of betrayal, a feeling that what had happened was not fair, was not according to the way the contract was written up. Finally, there was an anxiety associated with the question, what next?

The phasing-out process of this unit actually extended over a long period of time, though its demise came very quickly. There had been several crises during the four and one-half years of the unit's life, but most of the participants did not take them seriously, as most did not question whether the unit would survive. At some point after four years, however, those involved began to sense the end. Their reaction to this probability can be compared with that of people's reaction to a dying person. As it becomes evident that an individual is dying, the people about him begin to withdraw, and their behavior indicates that they know he is going to die. So, too, with this unit—demoralization set in and the staff started to scatter. They wanted to get out before the situation worsened. Many felt that it was a foolish and wasteful expenditure to invest any new energy in a dying program.

This was all it took to set off a chain reaction. The less energy people invested in the unit, the greater the acting out of hostilities such as blaming and scapegoating; the more openly hostilities were expressed, the faster the breakdown of the unit. One can say that the unit's death throes really began with the collapse of the idea of the group and with the lowering of morale.

How the Participants Saw and Explained the Unit's Death

The administrator of the hospital described the unit's death throes as he perceived them:

Rounds had been canceled for three weeks. I didn't know it, but the director had gone on vacation and no one else volunteered to sit in, so nothing much happened. The specialty therapist moved out. Then of course physical therapy got into the same thing and all of a sudden the director of nursing made a first thrust at closing the unit by going to the chief and saying that this situation was ridiculous. That's when it finally got to me, and I was told to look into it and see if the recommendation to close the unit seemed appropriate. The director made a feeble protest, saying that it was only because he was on vacation, that he could fill it right back up again. As a matter of fact, a week or ten days passed between when he said that and the time of the actual closing, and it didn't fill back up. There was no demonstrated concern about the unit until it reached such a point that there was little left to do there because there were so few patients. The staff were getting bored enough to make comments to their superiors, and the superiors were getting concerned about the waste of productivity because there were no patients there.

When asked if he thought he could have affected the outcome of the unit, he replied:

It would have happened on exactly the same date. I simply agreed it wasn't reasonable to let the place run with nine beds at that staff level. I agreed with moving the social worker from there. I had personally moved the specialty therapist from there, and the physical therapists were wasting their time for the same reasons. There was no medical support at all except for the director's, and I don't think that was enough to keep it running. Nursing had proposed a plan whereby they would make it a more generally orthopedic clinic. We could put a rehabilitation patient there tomorrow and have the therapists and the social worker come up, except that they couldn't be assigned there full time unless the need grew again. Nursing came up with a plan to shift the staffing around so that it wouldn't be as costly to run, given the fact there would be orthopedic and other kinds of patients who needed quite a bit of attention. The plan was passed right on through. I concurred with it. That was it.

The administrator, like others, advanced a critical view of the director's leadership role.

I think that it was a good enough unit so that somebody dynamic could have made it run and kept it full. But not this director, he was not the one. Whether it was simply because he was not dynamic enough or because his patient load declined too much, I don't know. I suspect that it was partly because there were too many physicians on the staff who would not refer patients to the unit because of the director.

The director of the unit was not initially consulted about whether the unit should be closed or continued. He was particularly unhappy about it. He was aware that hospital administration was displeased with him; he had the strong feeling that he did not have their support, but he had no idea why. He did state, "I think probably hospital administration would have liked to have seen a young person take over rehabilitation on this campus, somebody who would really push and develop a new program." In fact, the administrator would indeed have liked a more charismatic leader, but he had no new program in mind.

That the director was not consulted about the closing is an example of a common occurrence. The status of a leader changes when the organization he directs is in trouble; he is labeled a "lame duck," and at some point he is excluded from discussions. A conspiracy develops. Meetings are held by the higher leadership, from which the unit leader is excluded, and the fate of the leader or the fate of the unit, or both, are decided. Often, the leader first learns of changes through rumor. Sometimes, he is the last to hear that his fate has been determined or what his fate will be. He might hear a vague report from the chief of another department that some space currently occupied will soon be available, or a nursing director might state that some changes on the rehabilitation unit are anticipated, or a physical therapist might mention having heard that there would be a new director. By the time the leader is consulted, the decision has already been made, though protocol insists that he be offered the opportunity to go through a ritual in which he can try to defend his unit and plead for its survival. Although the doors to the unit are, in effect, closed, the higher levels of administration leave a slight crack in these doors, a crack the director could widen if he could convince the administration that they should not close the unit because of major risks or disruption involved in doing so. However, in this instance the arguments of the director were not heeded, and the decision that had been made without consulting him was implemented.

After the unit was terminated, the leader reevaluated his expectations and related his feelings about his role on the unit:

> I had wanted to be the director of it. But I would have appreciated it if somebody, whether my chairman, the dean, the chancellor, or the hospital administrator had come to me and said, "Joe, the way you're operating it is just not working out. How would you feel if we brought in somebody else?" I would have been perfectly happy to go along with something like that because my main interest was to keep the rehabilitation unit going. . . . My system is different than somebody else's, so that somebody else might be successful where I would fail. I look at it that way.

For the head nurse, the death of the ward coincided with the climax in her leadership struggle with the director, as she had heard second-hand that the budget had been reduced to nothing.

We were never even notified that the budget had been cut. I guess the director got the letter, or not even the letter, just the list of the amounts of money, and there it was—a big fat zero. I found out about it from someone else, but I had no idea how long it had all been in the works. This was really a shock to me. It was some time in January that I found out, and the director at the time wasn't going to do anything about it. Now whether he knew anything or not, I don't know, but the physical therapist and the social worker and I went to him and talked to him about it.

The head nurse attributed the unit's failure to lack of support for her actions. In particular, she placed emphasis on "the director, because he was not an efficient administrator. He wasn't aggressive or dynamic enough to really keep the place going." She thought he lacked the support he needed from the other medical staff. From certain persons, there came "disrespect and dislike, polite sarcasm and snide remarks, but always in a very polite way," a kind of high-class back-stabbing, according to her.

Repeatedly, the head nurse returned to the leadership problem, without focusing on the unique needs of this ward.

I think most importantly, if we had had a really strong leader, we would have been able to keep going. The teaching budget would never have been cut. It probably would have been increased if we would have proven that we really needed it. He couldn't. We really needed that budget. We would have had a house staff of our own—physical medicine and rehabilitation residents. We then could have had more patients, and the continuity of care would have been improved. A house staff would have been better for us, that is, the staff. Maybe I'm contradicting myself, because if we had a strong leader we probably would not have needed the house staff to give us the support we needed. As it was, we didn't have any support from anyone except each other.

She did recognize, however, that many of the unit's problems were augmented by the shortness of time that residents spent on the ward and by their general attitudes toward the unit.

We went through this two-month rotation bit, it was awful. The fellows were "putting in their time." They used that time to take their vacations and to do research projects, plus they were obligated to scrub both mornings when orthopedics had surgery. So these residents had patients on other floors besides their rehabilitation patients. We were just something they had to put up with.

She also felt that the hospital administrator lacked the kind of "toughness" or strength she thought a leader required.

I didn't think he was a strong person in saying the unit had to close. He was very supportive of the unit the entire time it was open. I felt he helped us a great deal in many ways. He got us more equipment, and he paid for the trip that four of us took to another hospital ward when no one else would pay for it. I mean he got us the money from administration. But he could see the handwriting on the wall when we'd have two and three patients and some weekends, no patients at all. To keep a unit open like that, you really are losing a lot of money. As much as I hated to see it close, I could certainly understand it. But I don't think that he was instrumental in insisting, or bringing it up to the administration.

While highly and vocally critical of the ward director, the head nurse felt no better equipped to take on the role of organizational leader than the director whom she condemned.

I just couldn't fight all alone and I wondered if it was really worth it. So I stopped. The whole four years it seemed to be a big battle, and I don't mind fighting if I can see that I can change something or that what I'm working for, fighting for, is really worth it. But it got to the point that it just wasn't anymore. We didn't have a resident, the director was almost nonexistent around here. . . . I quit.

She added how frustrated she was and how even the rounds did not provide the direction she needed.

I guess we'd need psychiatric rounds for support—someone to scream at or to blow off steam or whatever. I remember a few times when I certainly needed help and got it. I don't think that you can have a really effective rehabilitation program without an almost full-time psychiatrist.

While the head nurse was very open about her thoughts on the unit's demise, the auxiliary staff seemed reluctant to talk about its termination. None of them actually blamed any one person, although the director's failing were lightly touched upon. In the words of one aide:

We weren't really making any money. The patient should have been kept for a short period of time to teach him as much as possible using just a little of the budget and then we should send him home and let the family take care of him. I think the director could have applied himself a little more, maybe in other duties. When it got to the point where he didn't have any patients, then he should have gone out and sort of scouted around to see what he could find.

The reasons leading to the actual termination were not easy to define. Generally speaking, the participants tended to blame single individuals or units of people. Most perceived the failure in light of their own role in the picture. For example, the director was more concerned with people outside the unit, that is, the hospital administration, than he was with the "lower" staff or even the patients. The head nurse, on the other hand, though aware of the numerous challenges to running the unit successfully, focused the blame on the director and his personality (not his training, however). For the most part the participants failed to see the unit as a whole with many systemic vulnerabilities to which each member contributed and that each member had a major responsibility for overcoming.

Because everyone concentrated on everyone else's shortcomings, no objective discussion of the unit's death ever took place, nor was the provision for such analysis written into the unit's organization. The feelings of contamination that plagued those involved prevented the kind of social and anthropological autopsy that might have probed the sources for the unit's failure and might have diagnosed methods for preventing future failures. Such a discussion would also have alleviated the personal feelings of inadequacy that abounded, because it would have demystified the phenomenon of failure.

Just as the depression an individual feels when he fears failure often becomes a self-fulfilling prophesy, because the despondency itself shuts the person away from those who might help him, so the silence and sullenness that fell upon this unit toward its end precluded any possible saving analysis. Those involved feared that analysis would produce only mud-slinging, rather than have a beneficial effect.

There is a built-in tendency for nonprofit organizations to dismiss the failure of a project as though it were a machine that had broken down and was not worth fixing. Because the money it loses is not its own, a nonprofit organization does not feel the same pressure to analyze the causes of failure that an organization using its own funds does. Fears of recrimination or bad publicity or profitless slander can then assume control and keep any rational or systematic investigation from taking place. The result is a residual feeling of guilt and depression on the part of those involved, a twinge of shame in those tangentially connected with the failure, and a discomfort on everyone's part when asked to speak of the unit at all.

Systemic Problems Affecting Function and Dysfunction

We have now examined how a systems approach works and the values of using it, and we have articulated and analyzed some of the systemic problems this unit faced. Some of the conditions under which the unit was created, operated, and phased out, with impact of these on the functioning or dysfunctioning of the ward, contributed to the unit's eventual demise.

Multifunction Unit. A medical unit in a university hospital has special problems of organization and operation that stem from having simultaneously to offer patient care, serve as a teaching facility, and provide research opportunities. There are built-in vulnerabilities to such a system, and they must be given careful consideration in planning and design.

This multifunction aspect had a number of implications for the unit. It posed serious difficulties in the selection of patients, as several needs had to be met at the same time: (1) the need to treat patients who required rehabilitation, (2) the need to satisfy the staff, (3) the need to provide students with interesting case examples, and (4) the need to be economically solvent; that is, to maintain full occupancy.

The multifunction requirement affected ward life in the staffing patterns. Rather than a permanent staff, a rotating system was instituted for physical therapists in order to serve educational needs. This not only affected the quality of patient care, but it also interfered with the development of a sense of community and team effort among the staff.

The multifunction nature of the unit also created problems in staff relations and communication. Grand Rounds, for example, was expected to fulfill a multitude of often conflicting needs, and it was rarely able to do so.

Physical Setting. That the space for the unit was given to the planners already designed and complete jeopardized the success of the unit in that it probably kept the planners from conceptualizing fully the ways they expected the unit to function. Rather than being allowed to design a unit tailored to the needs of rehabilitation patients, planners were forced to alter their program to fit the physical realities of the unit.

The unit's small size proved to be particularly troublesome. Because rehabilitation requires such a large number of personnel, and because the running of a unit of whatever size must be on a twenty-four-hour basis, the nine beds of this unit quickly led to a disproportionate staff-patient ratio that made the whole endeavor appear extravagant.

Status of Rehabilitation Medicine. Several of the unit's problems were related to the specific status of rehabilitation as a field of medicine and as a treatment process. As it was a relatively new field, trained personnel were few and there was not yet a highly developed professional identity. There were few precedents for a hospital rehabilitation unit, making it impossible to benefit from another's experience.

Rehabilitation was not a popular specialty and thus did not attract the highest-quality residents or nurses. It was further isolated by differences in values between its treatment process and those of most medical units.

The variety and number of personnel required to meet a rehabilitation unit's needs created many difficulties. Such a large and interdisciplinary staff would be a challenge for any leader to orchestrate.

Finally, the chronic, almost hopeless nature of the patients' problems placed much strain on the staff's own morale. To remain hopeful and to feel that one's work is worthwhile when signs of improvement are so small and slow in arriving are feats requiring sometimes an overwhelming input of energy and dedication.

A Specialty Unit. Because the rehabilitation unit did not accept all types of patients, it was vulnerable to low census, yet for such a unit to succeed, the demand rate would necessarily have to be high. If the demand rate were too low, the unit would have to be filled with nonideal cases just to remain in operation. NIC (evaluation) patients were nonideal types on this ward, and their increased acceptance both added a new function to an already multifunction unit and created a sharp division in the needs and nature of the patient population.

Hospital Policy. New policy regarding the rights of staff made it impossible for a leader to hire and fire at will. The unit, therefore, became helpless in the face of dysfunctional workers, having to try to maintain staff unity and a high standard of patient care when some of the staff were incompetent. The leader's inability to force poor-quality staff to leave the unit added an aura of frustration and demoralization to the unit atmosphere.

Overlapping Administrative Control. The multiple authorities involved with the administration of the unit contributed to a blurring of principles and goals that, in turn, produced a tentativeness among staff who did not know which set of values to follow. The sense of unit autonomy and the development of a team concept suffered severely from having too many authority figures.

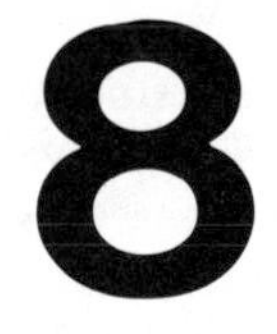

Success and Failure: The Role of Planning and Evaluation

Measuring Success

Several areas must be considered when evaluating a rehabilitation unit, or any therapeutic unit, for that matter. First, the nature of the particular patient population involved must be understood. Rehabilitation patients are, by definition, chronic or long-term patients. By the time they arrive on the rehabilitation unit, they have already gone through the acute phase of their illness elsewhere, perhaps on an orthopedic or a neurosurgical ward. For the most part, the rehabilitation ward receives only those patients who have not and probably will not recover completely from their illness. The man who fractures his hip and is put on an orthopedics unit where rehabilitation personnel teach him to use crutches and exercise is, after a period of time, discharged and expected to complete his recovery at home. He never sees the inside of a rehabilitation ward. Only when there is a promise of chronicity does the patient become a candidate for the rehabilitation unit. Because the initial condition of the patient threatens chronicity, the success rate on a rehabilitation ward will be necessarily lower.

Also, it is essential to define what we mean by the word "success." "Success" is a relative term and we must be vigilant against imposing such unrealistic goals on a rehabilitation program that a successful treatment becomes, by definition, impossible. In a sense, we must contradict something the American culture has taught us. We must learn to see success in gradual or incremental change rather than just in dramatic improvements. Americans love dramatic or grand metamorphoses–the ninety-nine-pound weakling who becomes Mr. Universe, or the three-hundred-pound failure who is now a curvaceous size "10" and a social success–and the medical environment is as vulnerable to these cultural pressures as any other group. We hear of sudden and painless cures, of a person who was crippled but who now flies an airplane or dances, of the tranquilizer that performs miracles. Failure is the monster behind the closet door; while we see success as a process that can be more or less understood, we neither discuss nor understand failure as a process.

This expectation of dramatic change is obviously incompatible with the state of the rehabilitation patient, for he is by definition a patient who does not recover. The conflict between the desire for quick and significant change and the realities of the rehabilitation patient's condition caused one of the major problems on the ward. Staff and patients and their families tended to dismiss as insignificant those small increments of improvement that did take place. Many did not believe, for example, that a 100 percent increase in function of a person with 5 percent function was worth achieving. From a strictly economical perspective, this might be arguable, but the rehabilitation unit was not created for economic purposes. Culturally, however, staff's notions of success also conflicted with the realities of rehabilitation possibilities, thereby damping any appreciation for or enthusiasm about what could be achieved. Because of this attitude, the extent to which the rehabilitation process would be considered successful by others was also minimized.

An American cultural attitude that causes further trouble for rehabilitation patients is that of believing only external incentives will move a person to exert serious effort. We do not see people as either inherently or self-motivated. Rather, we see them as the proverbial mules who must have a carrot stuck in front of their noses, always beyond their reach. In sales organizations, for instance, quotas are always set a little above what a person can expect to achieve. Anyone who sells over his quota will have the quota reset so that he must then achieve so much more in order to be successful. If he does achieve that so much more, he will still be only momentarily successful, for his quota will be reset again. Always there is the fear that if goals are put within easy reach, people will not do their best. Certainly, high goals can give a valuable impetus toward achievement, but we must be wary of goals that are unreasonably high. There is a fine line between the satisfaction and pride that come from hard work and a goal reached, and the frustration that arises from feeling that no matter how hard one works, the desired carrot will never be a jot nearer the mouth. Many patients on this rehabilitation ward felt that they were in a "catch-22" situation when it came to family, staff, and, indeed, their own goal expectations. If they did not work hard, the goals would almost seem within reach, but as soon as they really tried, the goals would jump higher and would be farther away than they were in the beginning.

Superstition, as much as we may wish to deny its force, is deeply ingrained in American culture, and there is a pervasive feeling that to say one will never be able to do something is to invoke evil spirits that will take that pessimistic statement and turn it into reality. "Think positively" or "Think big" or "Never say never"—all of these cliches are designed to exorcise the evil demon and call up the spirits of success. That there is an inherent difficulty in this attitude is obvious. There are things that cannot be done, accomplishments that cannot be achieved, and, particularly in rehabilitation programs, these limits, these areas of necessary failure, must be recognized and incorporated into the program.

Success and Failure of the Rehabilitation Unit

Keeping in mind the difficulty of evaluating the success of therapeutic units in general and rehabilitation units in particular, we can try to evaluate realistically the success of this rehabilitation ward.

The unit undoubtedly was quite successful in rehabilitating patients physically. It called upon all of the treatment innovations available at the time and used these to their fullest capacity. The unit was far from successful, however, in helping patients adapt to their social environment on the unit or in preparing them for integration into the community once they left the ward.

There were many reasons for the unit's failure in its social responsibilities. Economically, the social work time that was alloted did not allow for the kind of research necessary to investigate post-ward environments. A larger budget allocation for those professionals (either the social worker or the behavioral scientist) whose task is to go out of the unit and explore community attitudes and community facilities would have been necessary. But, and this is a second reason for the unit's failure to provide sufficient psychosocial rehabilitation, the unit leadership was not aware that a behavioral scientist should be called in for such a job. Whenever behavioral-science principles were introduced, they came via the channel of psychiatry rather than through sociology, anthropology, or social psychology. As a result, the professional resources that could have made a thorough social study of the patient's prospective environment were never utilized.

Because one of the few relief mechanisms available for inpatient residential staff comes with knowing that every case, no matter how long and how difficult, will have an end, little effort was made at follow-up, once patients left the ward. This also meant that the patient received minimal assistance in working out a self-help program for continued development after entering the community. The fact that no one person was responsible for continuity of care after the patient was discharged and the fact that it was often physically, economically, and geographically impossible for the staff to plan for anything beyond where the patient would be placed the day after he left the unit added to the difficulties in properly preparing the patient for his place in society.

Finally, and perhaps most importantly, the staff was unable to help in a patient's social adaption because the staff themselves often could not imagine that the patient could actually be successfully integrated into the community. In general, the staff did not have much optimism about their patients' futures. Instead, a kind of core depression pervaded the rehabilitation unit. The other side of overselling success was the underbelief, the sad, hopeless feeling staff had about patients. Expressed in many ways, this was the feeling that "if I were in your shoes, I wouldn't be trying hard. I wouldn't care enough to try to make life worthwhile, to learn how to bowl in a wheelchair, so to speak; because, if I were in a wheelchair, I wouldn't learn how to bowl—I'd blow my brains out, or something." It is hard to know how much of this despairing attitude was communicated to the patients; it is even harder to know how these thoughts could be eliminated from a rehabilitation ward; but it is hard not to conclude that such thoughts had a detrimental influence in the amount of attention paid to a patient's future outside of the ward.

On the whole, psychiatric effort on the rehabilitation unit was successful in dealing with immediate problems–in reducing extremes of behavior in patients, in helping staff to interact with patients, and in helping both to understand some of the psychological problems that might be involved. However, there was neither adequate time nor a favorable attitudinal environment for the psychiatrist to work on core psychological problems of either patients or staff. Basically, the psychiatrist encountered patients in crisis and staff in crisis, and in only a few instances did the psychiatrist do any follow-up counseling with patients after discharge. In fact, very few patients were referred to psychiatrists after they left the rehabilitation unit. This should seem odd, and it raises an important point. When a physical problem is great enough, as it always is in a rehabilitation case, we often fail to see that there is a psychological problem as well. Because each rehabilitation patient had sufficient physical reason to behave aberrantly, we neglected to probe for possible psychological problems.

The Planning Environment

The benefits of using a systems approach in evaluating any organization were emphasized earlier. A systems approach is also an ideal way of planning and designing an organization. This is particularly true when designing a unit like the rehabilitation ward, where people cannot be discharged once they are within the system. If one has the option of hiring and firing at will, it is not always necessary to consider all the possible ramifications of a system. A man opening a medical office, for example, is generally able to hire and fire whom he wants when he wants, and therefore need not necessarily consider ahead of time the space, the people he is going to require, the smoothness with which they will interact, or what their dissatisfactions will be. Those who will not have the freedom to discharge a troublesome worker must think more carefully before selecting workers. This careful planning involves a systems approach.

Systems thinking, however, requires a great deal of involvement and investment, far more than most planners give. Because planners of an enterprise usually are not investors in it, and because they will not be present when the system is functioning either poorly or successfully, they can afford not to take the time necessary to do more thorough planning. It would help, then, if as often as possible, planners of a system also be investors in it, so they will either benefit or have to take blame for what they plan.

Of course, a systems approach does not guarantee success and a nonsystems approach is not a promise of failure. Even experienced, profit-making organizations design enterprises that fail, with or without a systems approach. But, as a rule, unless a systems approach is adopted from the outset, one will progressively have to amputate certain parts of the system and graft on others to compensate for what was not originally thought of and for what does not fit.

A beginning step toward improving the planning of any unit is to understand the attitudinal environment in which the planning takes place. Planning committees tend to operate with different rules, depending on the source of funding for a proposed project, that is, whether the program is being federally funded or internally funded. When a project is to receive federal funds and when the program planning committee is composed of people from the same department, an atmosphere is generally created that discourages any question-raising. Individuals are requested to propose ideas that will add to the prospects of receiving a grant, but critical comments or proposals to shift resources within the existing organization are neither encouraged nor welcome.

When, however, a project is proposed that will be funded by the organization itself, usually by an internal shift of resources, then questions abound. Not only must the proposed change be strongly defended on its own merits but a convincing case also must be made for shifting resources from other programs. The unit that would have to surrender space, funds, or personnel is seen as the victim, deserving of sympathy or protection, much as though it were facing an invader or thief.

Once there is agreement on the objectives of the project and once it has been determined how the funds, space, and personnel will be acquired, the rules of discussion then shift. A "gentleman's agreement" is entered into that planning will be in the hands of those most directly concerned and that outsiders will offer only the broadest of suggestions. Specific suggestions or searching questions will now be considered an invasion of another's territory. It becomes exceedingly bad form to raise questions about what criteria will be used to decide when a unit has failed to reach its goals and should therefore be closed, its operations reduced, or its leadership and staff changed.

We might say that planning committees share the superstition we ascribed to patients, staff, and families earlier in this chapter. Any discussion of the possibility of a unit's failure creates anxiety that the conversation alone will in some way predispose the program to fail. No one likes an ill wish, and we have observed members of decision-making bodies knock on the table (wood) when the prospect of failure was discussed. Anyone who predicts failure in an atmosphere such as this not only casts doubt on the judgment of those who are predicting success but is also judged a pessimist and therefore a "loser." Any member who risks the disapproval of the group must have strong convictions and firm principles, particularly when he is jeopardizing nothing of his own.

Obviously, approaches to planning in such a setting are inadequate and irrational. While they may serve the interests of a few involved parties, they can in no way be seen to foster a high standard of care or maximum utilization of available resources. If we wish to provide optimal training and treatment facilities, we must organize planning committees less inclined toward cliquishness, defensiveness, and superstition and more ready to undertake the objective and thorough evaluation of a project. We urge, therefore, that planners become cognizant of those built-in factors that impede the planning process.

Planners in Medical Organizations [49, 50]

A second important step toward improved planning is the placement of planning responsibility into the hands of groups who are involved but are themselves outside the system and who are trained in general systems theory. There is ample evidence that planning a unit requires skill and knowledge in organization, but few who plan or design such units are social engineers or specialists in the field of organizational design. Rather, those who traditionally establish medical units are specialists in medicine, nursing, rehabilitation, surgery, and hospital administration. Because they are specialists, they seldom have a clear concept of the structure, function, or dynamics of an organization, nor do they have specifically delineated ideas of their goals or how their objectives are to be established, maintained, or revised. It is not their business to understand these concepts; it is the business of professional planners. Because these amateurs tend to overlook potential problems or defer planning for them and because their understanding of how to build an organization is limited, rehabilitation or any other units they design suffer the consequences. Such units frequently function with only partial efficiency, provide insufficient services for their patients, and create an unhappy working environment for the staff. Like a bad marriage that serves neither the spouses nor the offspring, rehabilitation and other medical units can continue along haphazardly for many years.

Using physicians or medical personnel as unit planners is not practical for a second reason, and that is that their attitudes toward designing usually are formed on the model of private practice. All too frequently, they apply private-practice guidelines to the designing of a unit. When physicians start private practices, they seldom do much long-range planning. They arrange for space, equipment, and assisting personnel, but most tend to underestimate what they will require. As they assume that patients will come to them in the same mysterious way that patients find other physicians, they make no contingency plans for failure. In fact, for the reasons already mentioned, the possibility of failure is never confronted. This lack of system usually works adequately in individual private practice, because the physician has the freedom to change almost any aspect of his operation at a moment's notice. If his practice declines, he can lay off staff; if it prospers, he can add to his employees. If he decides to end his practice and accept a salaried position, he need consider only his own desires; there will be no protesting outcry from any pressure group. All of these elements create an atmosphere in which detailed planning is unnecessary.

However, the physician planner will unconsciously bring some of his private-practice attitudes to conferences on designing university hospital units, and the hospital unit does not have the same flexibility. A university hospital ward is constrained by members of other professional roles, and it is subject to continuing audit by members of academic departments, clinical departments, and trainees. The freedom to move without having to answer to or be watched by others, which is typical of private practice, is not applicable to a hospital unit. Only the chancellor or the dean has the authority to open or close a unit, shift personnel, or redistribute resources, and in practice this tends to be accomplished only slowly. Furthermore, unlike private practice and even unlike profit-making hospitals, a medical unit in a university hospital has special problems of organization and operation stemming from the battle for emphasis between patient care, teaching, and research responsibilities.

An outside observer-planner is needed also because the physician-planner or administrator-planner will not be able to view the organization objectively. The difficulties involved in being a participant, an observer, and an administrator all at the same time should be apparent. Because, for example, the administrator is forced to make "yes-no" decisions, he necessarily must ignore certain valid considerations. A decision involves, by nature, the rejection of alternative but also valid considerations; that is, if there were no reasonable alternatives, there would be no decision to be made but only an action to be carried out. Because he must reject some possibilities in favor of others, the administrator-planner often will take a defensive posture and claim that his choice was the only possible solution and that, in fact, there was no real decision involved. Because of the difficulty in admitting to an inquirer, "Yes, those were other valid possibilities, but I chose these instead," the administrator-planner is not usually the person best qualified to analyze and then design his own unit.

A continuing problem an administrator will confront in attempting to analyze his own unit centers around his intense awareness of the individual personalities involved. He often attributes the success or failure of a whole system to the positive or negative aspects of personalities—either his own or others'. He may place the blame on his own lack of leadership or his lack of charisma; or he may feel that the fault lies with the poor attitude of his staff members or their lack of cooperation. Similarly, he may claim that success was due to the benign actions of one individual or to the cooperation of another or to his own skill in managing the unit. Because he sees discrete packages of decisions and actions and because he is involved with individuals, the administrator will find it difficult to think of the whole organization as a system of which he is only a part.

The extent to which this is true will be dramatically demonstrated should an administrator step out of his role in the system (as did the senior author of this book), stay out for a while, and then return to it as an outside observer. He will see his old role in a very different light. He will see what he could have done but did not do; he will become aware of many new possibilities he could not then see because he was locked into certain tracks; and he will be able to see the unit from other perspectives, getting a sense of how the unit functions as a whole.

Because of the limitations to which traditional planners are subject, we recommend that two distinct groups be commissioned to plan a unit, specifically, to plan a rehabilitation unit: (1) a group to handle the material aspects of the unit, and (2) a group to work with the interpersonal aspects of the unit. These groups would have different investments, skills, and interests, and they should exist simultaneously. The group considering the physical aspects of the unit would acquire and assign the space, deciding how it will be subdivided [14, 51, 52]. The second group would handle the interpersonal aspects of the organization, planning for human-relations problems before they flare up and can no longer be avoided. This is the group that never comes into being, and we will focus this discussion on it.

This group should deal with the qualitative aspects of a proposed program and should include behavioral scientists, particularly medical anthropologists. It should study the initial logistic plan and make predictions about the kinds of human problems that will probably occur if the group is allowed to evolve spontaneously. It should set up a series of hypotheses, recommend a series of interventions to test the hypotheses, and provide a set of alternate interventions should the initially recommended ones prove ineffective. This group should also plan and recommend techniques for maintaining the health of the organization.

The establishment of standards for evaluating treatment would also be one of the functions of the human-relations planning group. Such standards should specify the kind of care that will be given and the procedures for giving it. Since many disabled patients in a rehabilitation environment can achieve no improvement in functioning, the standards of treatment must be based on care rather than on improvement. Every rehabilitation unit should plan long-term follow-up procedures in order to evaluate treatment, and each unit should know the outcome of its own efforts so it can improve with subsequent patients. Such follow-up procedures might involve enlisting community support or contacting the patient's family. In any event, these procedures should be considered in the initial planning stages.

The human-relations planning group should also be responsible for designing a unit in which individuals can grow. This requires attention to in-service training and to the individual needs of the employees, and it should consider the potential destructiveness of supervisory pressures designed to improve performance. The group must also tackle the problem of fostering role and professional development while at the same time preventing the divisiveness and disintegration that can occur when professional roles are self-developed [53].

Keeping an Organization Healthy

In order to survive, a medical organization must not only achieve its primary goals for patient care, it must also provide for its own health [54,55]. To maintain the health of an organization, we must have a full understanding of what it needs, and we must build a healthy system to begin with [56]. This, of course, demands good planning, the anticipation of inevitable problems, and the prevention of problems that are not inherent.

A systems approach to the planning and evaluating of therapeutic units will require planners to anticipate the needs of the system, to:

(1) provide for a range of personality and functioning patterns,
(2) maintain a set of consumers,
(3) provide a method to identify and solve health and dysfunctioning problems both of the unit as a whole and of the individuals in it,
(4) maximize the functioning of the unit members,
(5) provide means for adapting to change, and
(6) select good staff to begin with.

Each of these areas will be considered in greater detail, noting obstacles to meeting the listed goals and possible ways of overcoming the obstacles.

(1) Provide for a Range of Personality and Functioning Patterns: One element that must always be considered in planning an organization is the personalities of which our organization will be composed; each human component in a system will have an individual personality. Although we can make certain judgments about a prospective team member's personality when we are recruiting personnel, we must keep in mind that all personalities have a range that rarely is apparent at the moment of recruitment. Some organizations try to get a better indication of this range by engaging in stress interviews, but this is generally frowned upon as unfair and inhumane and, as a result, it is rarely used in the selection process. The range of personality will determine the range within which a unit will function effectively. Much as a person building a machine would ask himself, "Under what temperature conditions will this machine function at full capacity, and under what conditions will it function at all?" the planners of a rehabilitation or other therapeutic unit must ask themselves a similar question about personality. It can then be gauged that within a certain boundary of stress and conflict, the unit will continue to operate maximally, but that once it crosses those boundaries in either direction, the unit will cease to function effectively and, eventually will cease to function at all.

(2) Maintain a Set of Consumers: There must be sufficient demand for a rehabilitation or any other unit to justify initiating the program, and this demand must be maintained at a level to sustain its operation. Planners, therefore, must provide effective means of measuring and encouraging demand. We will invoke the systems approach to understand and anticipate demand, for the systems approach forces planners to consider the implications of demand for the consumer and the requirements of demand for the service-giver. Unlike those less comprehensive assessments of demand that ask a prospective consumer, "Would you use

such and such a service were it available?" and then take the answer as a sufficient indicator of the demand, a systems approach requires that the implications of a new service to a potential consumer be analyzed. Questions such as, "How would a consumer have to change his life-style or professional work-style because of a new service?" or "How would the new service change a physician's relationships with his patients?" must be asked, because all of these factors ultimately determine whether a consumer's positive response will actually materialize into the kind of continuous use that a new service will require in order to maintain its operation.

This is particularly necessary when designing a specialized unit like the rehabilitation unit, for there is a finite number of potential consumers. The physicians who refer patients to the unit must continue to refer them or the program cannot survive. The rehabilitation unit of this study is a good example of a program that could not continue operations with the limited number of referrals it received. It needed a larger group of consumers, and to reach a larger group, it needed to do more public-relations work.

An advertising company that believed a good product will sell itself would soon go broke; such companies understand the dynamics of selling and would never operate on such a naive principle. Neither should a therapeutic unit. Someone must go out and actively present the positive aspects of the program—do a selling job, in effect.

(3) Provide a Method to Identify and Solve Health and Dysfunctioning Problems: An organization must be prepared for the health problems that inevitably will occur within the group. Health planners must realize from the outset that physical, mental, and social health problems will develop in any new facility among patients who are not accustomed to living together and who have not acquired techniques to maintain their mental and physical health in the new environment. Planners must consider, for example, the aggression that will certainly be in evidence while positions and status are being vied for—human beings share with chickens their instinct for a pecking order. Planners must then expect and plan for the depression that will result among those who are disappointed, and they must plan for the kinds of destructive interactions that can take place between members of an organization. Warning signals must be set up, maintained, and monitored, to sound an alarm when signs of disharmony, dysfunction, and unwillingness or inability to perform assigned tasks begin to appear.

The health of the group is only as good as the health of its individual members, and an organization must have ways of ascertaining and then combating any health problems among its personnel. As it cannot amputate, it must treat. A program that evaluates the staff's physical and mental health would serve two functions: it would protect the staff from what they might pick up from the patients, and it would protect the patients from what might be communicated to them by the staff. This, when it relates to physical diseases, is not controversial. However, staff members are far more sensitive about any routine examination of their mental health. An organization does not usually need a psychiatrist to inform it when one of its members has become psychotic, but it does need some kind of mechanism that can effectively isolate a disturbed individual and study the sources of his behavior change. Someone must be designated to confront the staff person with those aspects of his behavior that are disrupting the organization and then analyze the explanation given. The alternative of individual therapy should be offered, to help the suffering staff person and to make sure that the disturbance does not spread to other parts of the organization. In a medical organization, the patient and staff must be protected at all cost.

To remain healthy, an organization must be able to replace or improve persons who are not performing. When it cannot, it operates with a diseased part, and much like a person who is physically ill, an organization with a dysfunctional worker seems to become depressed, irritable, and inefficient. The non- or poorly functioning worker, therefore, should be planned for in advance, before the problems arise. There are risks to firing such a worker, and there are risks to keeping him. Firing the worker indicates to others that the organization is unfeeling and will not adjust itself to help one of its members. But firing also indicates that an organization is firm in its requirements and standards. Firing, it must be noted, can also be costly if its impact on the worker produces some psychiatric disturbance that would make him eligible for workers' compensation benefits. On the other side, keeping a dysfunctional worker often implies that the organization is not firm in its requirements, and it tends to demoralize the rest of the staff. Keeping the worker can also create a situation in which scapegoating can flourish.

Finally, an organization, to remain healthy, must always monitor how it is using its members' potentials. *The Peter Principle* was written about people who attain positions that exceed their level of competence. The opposite problem, underutilization of ability, is also relevant. Members of a therapeutic environment who are not permitted to exercise the full range of their abilities or whose range of competence is not recognized become disenchanted, sometimes without even knowing why. They become angry and feel that the organization itself is not functioning maximally, an understandable reaction since the organization is not using the workers' potential, and they become critical of others, particularly those in authority who show weakness. In a situation like this, the organization loses in two ways: it loses because it does not fully utilize the human resources at its disposal, and it loses because it eventually forfeits even those resources it was using, the worker having become depressed, angry, disillusioned, and nonfunctioning. As these are contagious feelings, they often spread to other staff members, even those whose capacities are being fully realized. A shadow of low morale falls over the unit, and no one knows why.

One important component of the therapeutic rehabilitation environment, therefore, will be a program that permits all members to grow by encouraging them to develop skills and techniques and by helping them to increase their knowledge. We might even assert that such a program should be required, and that each member of the staff should be not only encouraged but expected to fulfill his potential as a therapeutic agent. Instruction from peers, superiors, educational sources, and experiential learning situations all can be invoked to achieve this goal, and a provision should be written into the budget of each unit for resources to fund the program.

(4) Maximize the Functioning of the Unit Members: Dissatisfaction, confusion, and disenchantment with an organization can arise when staff members do not know before they walk onto the unit anything about what their job will actually be like. An orientation session should be designed to prepare the staff for what they will encounter. This will not be a simple task, however, because planners seldom know what to prepare the staff for. The fantasy about a unit, the way people imagine it, is often very different from the unit's reality. Staff members do not really know the personalities of the other people with whom they will be working, nor can the actual experience of an eight-hour day in the environment be known; and it is impossible to determine beforehand what the patients will be like.

One way to ease the uncertainty is to recognize at the outset that neither the director nor the nursing director nor the physical therapist really knows what the environment is going to be like. Everyone should be permitted, therefore, verbally to wander through the range of their expectations and so at least acknowledge them. They may then become aware before they begin the job of what some of their disappointments and some of their gratifications might be.

This should, in fact, be seen as a continuing process and, started early enough, it can become part of the culture of the unit. Discussions of expectations and resulting disappointments could prevent some of the anger, frustration, and sense of being cheated that so many staff members come to feel. We might call this a systems or group approach to satisfaction and dissatisfaction, differing from the individual or personality approach in which part of the group releases its dissatisfaction by blaming or scapegoating another member.

The preparation of flow sheets can help to orient staff to a new unit. Flow sheets simulate what might actually happen on the unit over an eight-hour period, and we can make the analogy between the use of flow sheets to prepare the worker for the demands of a therapeutic unit and the use of "war games" to prepare a soldier for battle. Even though the most intricate war games are only models, even though they may not reveal all of the problems or even 80 percent of them, they will at least alert those involved to the categories of problems they can anticipate. Like the sharing of expectations, flow sheets should be made a continuing part of the unit. This would help to emphasize the unit's functioning as a system and would lessen the pressure on individuals.

The personality needs of staff members must be considered if they are to perform maximally. While this runs contrary to the general view, it is impractical to think that personality needs can be ignored. Many people—employers, employees, patients, and children—are unwilling to acknowledge personality needs in another, particularly when there is a larger goal in sight. They want to think, instead, that a person needs only to decide what must be done and do it. In other words, they want to think that a person can function like a machine—constant, correct, and nondemanding. Consequently, they are intolerant of a person who fails to perform as he should, and they are unwilling to expend the energy necessary to bring the unhappy team member back into a working state. That people are not machines is obvious; that they will not perform well if they are treated like machines should also be apparent. Personality needs, from the lowest worker to the highest leader, must be acknowledged if the team is going to operate at peak efficiency.

Finally, every organization should have a system of rewards to let the staff know that it appreciates good work. Organizations like the Cub Scouts understand the importance of recognizing merit, and they reward their members regularly. Large organizations do the same, giving out service certificates and awards at regular intervals. Therapeutic units must also recognize the basic need to be rewarded for effort expended and time spent. By demonstrating satisfaction with workers, the unit will reinforce team members' desire to achieve by giving them incentive to do more.

(5) Provide Means for Adapting to Change: Every organization must expect and learn to tolerate change. Because change conflicts with the tendency of organizations to standardize behavior into fixed roles, the means for adapting to change must be provided at the organization's inception. Often it becomes apparent at some point after the organization has begun to operate that the initial role specifications must be modified. The organization, then, must have the flexibility to make those changes or it will cease to operate effectively. The flexibility to change the roles of team members, to augment, diminish, or exchange duties among them, must be built into the system from the start. If this flexibility is not written into the initial charter, the organization will have no means of adapting to unseen contingencies and will be at the mercy of every variable that appears [57].

(6) Select Good Staff to Begin With: Planning for the problem staff person is essential, but if the organization is to achieve its goals and retain the respect of outsiders, it initially must look for excellence in its staff. When selecting the excellent staff person, planners must consider personality as well as training. Frequently, those who are technically well qualified for a job prove unable to perform some of the subtle interpersonal aspects of the work, tasks that require sensitivity, compassion, and diplomacy. They can perform the specific parts of the job, the parts in which a person can be instructed, but they cannot relate to

other human beings in ways that will reassure and involve them. Some people, whatever their training, are unable to make decisions. Fear of criticism or obsessiveness about the "right" solution makes them incapable of performing administrative duties. Others with far less training may have no difficulty in analyzing and resolving problems. As it is through its staff that an organization will often make its strongest or weakest impression, it is essential that both the job requirements (technical and human) and the job applicant be carefully considered so that the best job-person fit can be made.

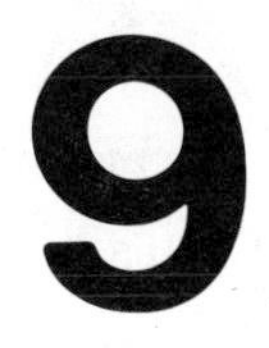

General Recommendations

The prospective leader of a rehabilitation unit needs a guide to the problems of decision-making, particularly for the type of unit we have described in this book, but we would be hard pressed to suggest an orientation and leadership program for most hospital units until they have first been studied. Certainly, we could not have predicted the nature and variety of this unit's problems if we had not interviewed each person on the unit and had not observed the ward members' interactions in many different situations. Such problems as the lack of admissions standards or the occurrence of sadistic relationships between staff and patients probably would not have been predicted when the unit began. Having made such a study, however, we are in a position to make recommendations for a unit similar to this one and for other small rehabilitation units that resemble it in leadership, personnel, and function.

Our first recommendation would be that each existing unit contract for an individual study, whenever possible. Some of the areas that must be considered are listed below, and recommendations are made for each area, on the basis of this study.

The physical setting

Roles

Leadership

Communication

Values: a "Culture of Care"

Staff functioning and satisfaction

Patient-staff relations

Psychosocial needs of the patient

Support systems

Budgeting

Community considerations

If a unit decides to contract for its own study, some of the questions that should be asked are:

Physical setting:

What facilities are necessary for the unit to function maximally?

What facilities are desirable for patient and staff welfare?

How does the space coincide with the needs of a unit?

How will people interact in this space?

Does the space allow both for privacy and company?

Roles:

How well-defined are the roles?

What provision has been made for altering any given role?

Do the roles fit the jobs?

Leadership:

Who is the leader?

What are the functions of the leader?

What is the relation of the leader to his superiors? To his subordinates?

Communication:

Should communication channels be formalized within the unit?

How do communication channels between the unit and the hospital and between the unit and the community function?

Values:

What are the primary goals of the unit?

What are the methods for enforcing these goals?

How is responsibility for enforcement to be assigned?

What is the unit's attitude toward individual staff development?

How will the unit relate to community needs and social values?

Staffing:

What types and numbers of staff will be needed?

What criteria should be used in selecting staff?

How can staff abilities be fully used and developed?

What morale problems can be expected to emerge, and how should they be handled?

Patient relations:

What is the patient's role on the unit?

Should there be guidelines prescribing staff relations with patients?

Should the physician be honest with the patient about the actual extent of the patient's disabilities and chances for improvement?

Budgeting:

How much support can realistically be expected?

What can be done to encourage community and other funding?

Community considerations:

Where should the unit be located?

How does the unit meet community needs?

These questions will be answered as they pertain to the rehabilitation unit of this study.

Physical Setting

A good rehabilitation ward design, in contrast to the one described in this book, would maximize the advantages of privacy found on this unit but also would provide space for both social and therapeutic activities. Patients and staff would be contiguous, but not necessarily together. A patient would be able to look out of his room and see movement and activity, but he also could be alone. Easy access to all facilities for all patients would be provided, and no special structures would be allowed to separate staff from patients. Different facilities would be provided for the various kinds of activities: a television room for those who want to watch television, a social room for those who want to talk or play cards, and a room where one can read undisturbed.

Most importantly, the design would recognize that the rehabilitation unit is the patient's home for a long period of time and, as such, it should have all the necessities of a home—including dining, cooking, and grooming facilities. Although any design must keep in mind that staff members have to work and treat patients on the unit, the focus should be on the patient and his needs. The patient must be made to feel that this is the best possible environment and that everything that can be done for him is being done. Since the patient spends relatively little time in physical-therapy activities, facilities for these purposes (swimming pool, for instance) need not be on the unit itself. Those facilities that will help the patient to convert the rehabilitation unit into his temporary home are of prime importance, and should be so considered in the design of the unit.

Roles

Those planning a unit like to think that the unit will be one large happy family and that an easy, relaxed cooperation that makes role boundaries unnecessary will emerge naturally. Because they feel that setting such boundaries explicitly will reduce the flexibility of the staff and produce hair-splitting about who should do what, planners are afraid to define role boundaries at all. Unfortunately, it is just this lack of role definition that creates the petty arguments the planners are trying to avoid.

Staff members themselves try to provide what the planners have left out and they create de facto definitions of their own role boundaries. As a consequence, they often refuse to take on tasks that would enable them to help other staff members. It is much easier for staff to cooperate with each other when the boundaries have been defined from the onset. A staff member can then willingly go beyond his prescribed role to help someone else, without fearing that the task will then become part of his regular role or that others will think he is overstepping his position. Just as the secure child who knows his present limits and is sure he will not be abandoned or pressured can more easily explore his boundaries than can the insecure child, so a staff member who knows how his role is defined can step outside to assist another without fearing that he will never get home again.

However, the initial defining of roles must not preclude alterations of those definitions [58]. Functions do change, and as an organization evolves, it often becomes apparent that the staff must be employed in different ways than those originally planned [59]. If those changes are presented unexpectedly to the staff, dissatisfaction, a slump in morale, and subtle or overt acting out can result, making the unit operate less effectively and thus depriving the patients of optimal care. Roles, therefore, should be redefined regularly, in the presence of all persons involved.

Administrators often are fearful that staff members will not be amenable to surrendering parts of their functions or to assuming new functions. A more optimistic view should be taken. If the staff have participated in the planning, development, and evolution of the unit, and if they are then called together to confront a new challenge that might involve additional work for many or all of the team members or that might entail sharing the work of an overburdened staff member, they usually will work out a plan to achieve the desired goal. The morale of a unit can be measured by how it meets a challenge such as this.

There must also be a structure or procedure for defining the sick role. All staff members should share similar expectations of what the patient is to achieve while on the ward and how he is to behave. If, as on the rehabilitation ward of this study, the director expects one kind of behavior from the patient and the head nurse expects another, the patient will have no guide for playing his role. In fact, as we have seen, the patient will be punished if he behaves according to the director's version of the sick role (staying on the ward as long as possible) and does not conform to the head nurse's role definition (quick achievement of independence). Staff members should not be permitted to create definitions of the sick role independent of each other, for this can have a harmful effect on rehabilitation. Because a severely impaired patient is not in a position to do much adapting, each staff member must be aware of any demands he makes on patients other than those agreed upon by the staff as a whole.

Leadership

To plan for the problems of leadership that might develop on a rehabilitation unit, the designers should examine available studies and make as much use as possible of the practical experience of others. Orientation sessions based on what can be learned should be given not only to the unit leaders but also to the entire staff.

There is much magical thinking in organizations, and those directing and controlling the organization avoid raising controversial issues because they fear that, by admitting the existence of potential problems, they will turn them into actual problems. Leaders tend to hope that somehow the organization will function smoothly if the dust, so to speak, is swept under the carpet. Needless to say, this can become a basis for conspiracy. Leaders are not forced to bring problems to the surface, and subordinates may well approve this willful blindness because they can then continue to function as they wish. Neither is forced to confront the areas of friction until the problems have become so large that cooperative effort is impossible. The only way this state can be avoided is by bringing all members of the staff together to participate in planning for and discussions of leadership problems.

Of the few choices available as leadership models, we would recommend basing the leadership of a small rehabilitation unit on the model of the family business. Unlike the rigid, fixed model that was used on the rehabilitation unit studied, a family business model would permit fluidity within the unit. The leader or leaders would have the obligation of helping the members grow to their maximum potential. Each member of the organization would be encouraged to advance and to undertake leadership responsibilities compatible with his experience. Guidance would be offered, and criticism would be constructive and educational rather than destructive. Within the limits permitted by law, each unit member would be encouraged to expand his role and to develop his skills to their fullest.

Leadership, under this model, would become a dynamic force—taking chances, permitting novices to try, recognizing and accepting failure. Such a leadership would also have to recognize that the fluidity of roles it fosters will make outsiders anxious. It also will make those within the structure anxious, for sufficient permissiveness probably will result in increased staff demands. Members who have tried and succeeded in new activities might challenge leadership and insist on greater participation. Members might even become more skillful at certain tasks than the leaders themselves, and they might then become critical of the leadership. Obviously, these risks are among the apprehensions that keep leaders from permitting role fluidity and experimentation with leadership functions. As a result, the tendency is usually toward following leadership models in which the roles are fixed, responsibility is assigned, and programs for accountability are established. This rigid leadership design in a health organization, however, leads to dissatisfaction on all levels and deprives the patient of the therapeutic benefits that would be available to him under a growth-fostering leadership model. This recommendation may seem to contradict earlier statements about the need for well-defined roles, but what is needed is role definition with fluidity—a kind of controlled chaos. Staff need to know what their roles are; this gives them stability and the courage to test their own potential. But they also need to feel that they can progress within a role, that their initiative and ambition will be rewarded. A leadership model based on the family business would allow for both of these patterns.

It is unlikely that such an organizational design will evolve unless it is planned specifically, although it does exist to some extent in all organizations. When such a model occurs spontaneously, it is usually the result of a special relationship between the leaders and the staff. Sometimes a particularly involved leader will foster the growth of a staff member, and sometimes an especially strong and talented staff member can push his way into a position of higher responsibility. Usually, however, this is not the case, and staff remain stationary within their assigned roles. We should caution, however, that if a family business model of leadership is to thrive, it must be understood and supported by all levels of the administration, which in the case of the rehabilitation unit would be both hospital and medical administrations.

Another important consideration in planning leadership concerns the sharing of responsibility. On a small rehabilitation unit, staff and patients must share with leaders responsibility for the actions of the group, and this sharing cannot be artificial. It cannot, for instance, consist of a series of notices that inform staff and patients of actions taken or about to be taken. Often those problems in which staff have a vested interest are problems that must be decided by the staff. Although from time to time the unit director or the leader of one of the subgroups on the unit will have to notify the staff of a decision that comes from above, the leader must present this decision to the group and inform them of their possible recourse, even if the only recourse is a letter of protest.

If leadership is to share responsibility with staff, then staff must also share responsibility with leadership, and staff members often are ambivalent about taking on responsibility. They often prefer the role of critic; the leader takes the initiative and they point out the weaknesses or faults. The staff must therefore be trained to participate in decision-making and in decision implementation. The leader cannot carry the whole burden alone, and it is as important for staff to share responsibility as it is for leadership to give them a chance to do so.

Leaders, while they share decision-making with staff, must be careful never to subvert the authority of the administration superior to them. They must never try to undermine their superiors' decisions. They can disagree openly and discuss their disagreement with staff. They can initiate and coordinate protests, but they must not take any steps that could fall into the category of "acting out." Although they may gain temporary approval and even affection from their staff by leading a revolution, they must remember that they are setting an example and that the same tactics may then be used by staff to undermine their own decisions.

Even when a leader has natural ability and is objective, there is need for external supervision. Medical organizations must have some kind of reviewing body that can say to the leader, "No, you can't just go ahead and do it this way; we insist that you resolve the situation or we'll step in. We are not going to permit a standoff to continue in these relationships, because this is not your organization. We are responsible for it. The rehabilitation unit doesn't belong to you, leader, or to you, head nurse, or even to the collective you and the patients."

Such strong supervision actually can help a leader to maintain the quality of a unit, for it warns the entire staff that standards are not the caprice of one person; they are part of a larger culture and will be maintained. The leader must be able to tolerate this kind of supervision, just as staff must tolerate supervision from him. He must recognize that he, too, is a human being who will not be seen as perfect at all times. This is a difficult position to maintain, for it involves recognizing his own fallibility while at the same time sustaining his role as leader of the unit. In effect, the leader must try to remain objective even though he is intimately involved.

Experienced leaders set limits to the fluid structure of their organizations very early; they recognize a range of behavior and of rights and, within these boundaries, they are willing to negotiate. The boundaries, however, are fixed. If the leaders find that they are being forced to submit in nonnegotiable areas, then they should be prepared to relinquish their leadership, and a change in leadership always has unpleasant ramifications–bad publicity, difficulty of finding a better leader, and a possible upset in the faulty but at least existing equilibrium.

Communication

Formal communication channels and the procedures for using them should be established very early in the development of the rehabilitation unit [60]. They should be carefully designed, and their use should be mandatory. It is not enough that they merely be available for use should the need arise, because people left to their own desires usually will postpone using the channels until too late.

Whether in a family or in a working situation, people will tend to avoid an intelligent, rational examination of controversial or problem issues. Each person is afraid that after he has stated his viewpoint, others will either withdraw from him or will retaliate. Often he is equally afraid that he will not be able to control his emotions and so will not be able to state his view in such a way that a hostile counterreaction can be avoided. As a result, he holds his objections or his unhappiness inside until the tension builds to such a degree that he blurts out his thoughts, overstates his views, and produces the very reactions he feared.

Established communication procedures should alleviate this problem, because an opportunity to raise dissatisfactions is provided before they become miseries or bitterness. Regular conferences can be used to teach the members of the team how to communicate with each other. While this is usually a slow process, it is highly educational, for it has the effect not only of teaching team members to communicate with each other but also of teaching them to communicate with patients and their families and with other persons concerned in the rehabilitation process.

Rounds are the major communication channels on a rehabilitation unit, and rounds can serve many different functions. The term "rounds" describes a formal discussion of several patients, but it does not define what is going to be discussed, how it will be discussed, who will direct the discussion, or who will participate in it. A constitutional procedure for rounds, specifying their particular functions, should be designed when planning the unit. For example, some units might find that they need three different kinds of rounds. Teaching rounds could be directed by a few staff members (residents, physicians, or nurses) who would be assigned to present an in-depth review of a patient's case, including literature bearing on the treatment, a diagnosis, and possible research opportunities. Planning rounds and treatment rounds could also be designed to serve particular patient needs and to work as channels for staff communication.

In planning these rounds, each detail should be considered in advance–who will talk, who will not talk, how much time each participant will be allotted for presenting his view. We must keep in mind, however, that the specifics of the plan will not be precisely applied. They will serve as a map and they will make boundaries known, so that when one person starts to ramble across the boundaries, he can be pulled back within the map area.

Likewise, there should be boundaries of protocol, a set of rules that dictates how people will interact. If each participant feels that he has the freedom to say whatever is on his mind, regardless of its effect on someone else, or if people feel that they can interrupt each other at will, the result can only be a chaos of ill feeling. There must be some sort of order, some rules to govern behavior, and while the rounds might be less spontaneous because of this, they will also be more productive as the participants will be forced to think, and think reasonably, before they speak.

Values: A "Culture of Care"

In planning a unit, it is essential that values be carefully defined. Otherwise, as we have seen from the example of this rehabilitation unit, the personal values of individual staff members will supercede any undefined values of the ward. A comprehensive treatment program in rehabilitation, one that attempts to create a "culture of care" will propose and discuss with the staff several basic ward values or functions of the unit.

The first component of a culture of care would be a conscious, stated agreement among all members of the staff and among the leadership that the care and welfare of the patient is the first priority [61], and that no other consideration will take precedence over this. Without doubt, almost every reader will agree to this value, claiming that it is understood, but we often forget the important difference between a tacit understanding of something and a stated agreement. In many medical institutions, attention to economic, research, or training principles overrides attention to the care and welfare of the patient. Although no one would willingly state this fact openly, it is stated often enough through action and practice, and the unwillingness to face the issue of priorities represents a silent conspiracy to divert energies from the patient-care goal. Because the primacy of patient care is not directly affirmed, we can expect that something less than an ideal or even viable culture of care will develop. There must be no excuses acceptable for subordinating this care to any other goal or value, and the agreement to place patient care above all other considerations must have a force like that of a constitutional amendment or a commandment. No departure from the stated agreement can be tolerated.

There also must be a firmly established and specifically articulated method for delivering care—how will care be delivered, how much care will be delivered to each patient, how often will care be delivered and by whom? Obviously, no exact program can be detailed for all patients; individual treatment regimens will be developed at admission and as the patient's therapy progresses, but unless the issue of quantity, kind, and quality of care is considered, it will be very easy to benefit one patient at the expense of another or to cheat all of what is rightfully theirs.

A sense of joint responsibility for the delivery of quality care must likewise be maintained. There can be no license to overlook poor-quality care because it is provided by a separate discipline. Each person in the therapeutic environment must be his brother's keeper and protect his coworker from slipping into shoddy habits and therefore giving the patient far less than he deserves and far less than the worker has to offer.

Further, there must be a programmed reaction to any departure from the standards of care. Anyone who is negligent or delinquent should be censured and should *feel* censured. There must be blame, and there must be shame, and there must be the invocation of guilt. The union of staff against patients in a therapeutic setting must not be allowed. It is all too easy for staff to commiserate with each other about the low pay or about some of the unpleasant aspects of the work or about lack of appreciation from many sources, including the patient. Such commiseration can only be deemed an excuse for giving the patient less than full care.

The responsibility for assisting and educating each therapeutic person must also be shared. Irrespective of where the formal responsibility for educating and training staff lies—with the physiatrist for physical medicine and rehabilitation staff, with the physical-therapy department for the physical therapists, with the nursing service for the nursing staff—each must also educate persons in other disciplines. No one service should be permitted to "own" people or assume sovereignty over them. No one service should be allowed to say, "We'll train ours and you train yours." Neither should the culture of the unit permit any one service to claim invasion when members of another specialty or discipline educate its members. In fact, the culture of the unit must insist that it is not only the right but the obligation of each service to educate members of both its own and other disciplines. The culture of care should not allow the kind of specialization, either of function or of education, that is demanded by unions or industrial and nontherapeutic service organizations.

Still another value that must be weighed against all those described affirms that society also has rights. Just because an individual has suffered some catastrophic injury does not automatically mean that he has the right to ten months or ten years on this rehabilitation unit. Other persons have the right to use this unit also. We must decide who has the right to this space and for what length of time these services should be permitted to continue.

Once a comprehensive set of values has been established, each staff member will be able to see what must be done in order to fulfill the goals of the correspondingly defined functions. All staff members working on the ward will be expected to devote their full time to the attainment of these goals. They will also be expected to cooperate with each other. No staff member should interfere with the work of his comembers. Instead, he should do everything in his power to further the effectiveness in serving the welfare of the patient. We do not ask that staff not complain; we ask that they not obstruct. Staff must also be circumspect in their communications to other staff members and patients, so that they do not introduce bias, error, or rumor into the system. Most importantly, staff will be expected to act in a professional role and to adhere to the ethics of the medical profession while at the same time following the ward values and helping to create a culture of care.

Improving Staff Functioning and Satisfaction

One of the first things we can do to help staff adjust to working on a therapeutic unit is to prepare them for the marked differences they may confront in that environment. We might look at the Peace Corps orientation process as an exemplary model. Before sending its members off to a foreign country, the Peace Corps teaches them a great deal about the culture they are going to encounter. The members are taught some of the culture's complexities, some of its symbolism, some of its idiosyncracies (from their perspective), and some of the ways it differs from the worker's own culture. The Peace Corps trains its members this way so that when the worker arrives in his new environment, he will not suffer from what anthropologists call "culture shock," and either fall apart or behave in a way that is offensive to the receiving group. In much the same way and for many of the same reasons, professionals going to work in special therapeutic units should be carefully prepared. The question then arises, prepared for what?

Most staff who will work on a therapeutic unit already will have had experience with the specific diseases or handicaps of the patients who will inhabit the unit, so they need not be briefed on how to handle the ailments themselves. Physical therapists will have worked with such patients in outpatient settings. Nurses will have worked with crippled people and with ill people in general; and all the staff will have worked with both the acutely and the chronically ill. The workers must be prepared for certain qualitative differences in working on a rehabilitation or other therapeutic ward, however [62]. All patients in this environment, not just one or two, will have the same problems; they will be on the ward for a long time; and there will be a high demand for personal services from the staff. This is in contrast to usual staff experience on other wards where patients are mostly ambulatory and, though ill and hospitalized for evaluation and treatment, generally are able to take care of many of their own needs. They can bathe themselves, for example, and feed themselves.

Staff must also be prepared to face their own reactions to the work conditions they will encounter. They must be prepared, for example, for the inevitable problems that will arise when working with severely disabled people for an extended period of time. One can tolerate almost any kind of difference in another human being if the encounter is brief enough; however, by increasing the duration of the encounter, we increase the amount and intensity of intolerance as well. Staff must be trained both to acknowledge this and to develop methods of compensating for their reactions. They should expect that, over time, their likes and dislikes of certain patients will intensify. Their fondness and affection for, and perhaps erotic feelings toward, some patients will grow stronger and, conversely, their irritation or antipathy toward other patients will also become more severe. An uncooperative patient on an acute service can be tolerated easily because he soon will be discharged. An uncooperative patient on a rehabilitation unit is another case entirely. The staff often feel the involvement will never end.

The staff person must also be reminded that patients frequently feel similarly about the staff. Just as certain quirks in a patient will irritate a staff member, mannerisms of the staff member may irritate the patient. All of the implications of a long-term stay apply to the patient as well as to the worker.

We must, therefore, sensitize staff to the kinds of traits that might become irritating to them. Differences in values and habits, as discussed earlier, are a fertile source of conflict between staff and patients. More specifically, differences in eating, grooming, and dress habits and differences in vocabulary or speech patterns (especially swearing) can be especially provocative.

The variety of the patients' social backgrounds must be considered, and the staff must be prepared to encounter a wide range in intelligence, education, and social status among the patient population. It may, for instance, be difficult for a nurse to tolerate someone who is of much higher social status; any sort of condescending or demanding behavior on the part of such a patient would take on a symbolic value it would not have were the patient of lower status. By taking the time to train the staff at the unit's inception for the kinds of frustrations and hostilities they probably will feel, we may sensitize them so that when they do encounter negative traits in a patient, they do not become overwhelmed and strike out at the patient, thus starting an antagonistic relationship that may be impossible to correct.

In a recent newspaper column, a writer suggested (tongue in cheek) that money should be given directly to the poor because so little of it is left after it passes through the bureaucracy. This suggests the unconscious and unquestioned tendency of governmental bodies that are established to serve some particular group, to end by serving themselves. In a bounded, walled therapeutic community, such self-serving tendencies are likely to occur because there is a greater measure of identification with the unit. On medical units, a staff "floats," members come and go, and they tend to identify with the larger nursing or specialty staff; on psychiatric or rehabilitation units, staff identify with each other and with the unit. A greater "payoff" therefore is necessary on these units, where the work is more demanding emotionally. The staff person must do more than his technical job; he must relate to the patients and to other staff members and actually become a part of the family. He must see the project as a team effort and he must make himself one of the team members. Just as we expect special rewards from the family we join, a staff member will expect to get more from his dedication to the unit than just his salary. The salary is for the work he performs; the loyalty, love, and emotional commitment invested must be rewarded also.

Consultants are special kinds of staff members, and perhaps the most important consideration regarding them is that, inasmuch as they can be chosen, they should be chosen very carefully. In many cases, staff are given to a unit and the unit is then, for good or ill, saddled with them. But a unit does not need to be burdened by inappropriate or inadequate consultants. Just as a family does not need a destructive friend when seeking help, so a therapeutic unit does not need a destructive consultant. They should be chosen carefully and strategically, and they should be changed when necessary.

To gain maximum use from their consultants, units must be clear about the role they want each consultant to play and they must articulate fully how that role might differ from one played on an acute care unit. The consultant should also be given some orientation to the specific goals and methods of the program. Some preparatory discussion with the consultant would help to avoid unwanted advice that would create stress for a patient or dissatisfaction among the staff. The unit must then try to incorporate the consultant into the team so that he does not seem to be a foreign element. If, after having prepared the consultant in these ways, he is unsatisfactory or it is found that he cannot be trusted to stay within the prescribed guidelines, then he should not be invited to consult a second time.

Patient-Staff Relations

We have already made a plea for honesty between patient and physician, and should emphasize again the necessity for openness when dealing with a patient. If the physician is not direct with his patient, then the staff will end by carrying the physician's burden. The staff themselves eventually will have to tell the patient the truth, and when this happens, the patient's attitude toward and motivation for improving may be seriously impaired.

If a patient is in a reasonably clear state of mind, the entire staff should discuss his status with him. They should tell him what his condition is, what his prospects for recovery are, and what abilities will be worth working for. He should be told the price he will have to pay and the limits he cannot expect to exceed. Because patients become highly sensitive to the reactions of staff and to staff's motivations for rehabilitating them, it is essential that staff examine their own feelings very carefully to avoid telling the patient that he will improve while covertly concluding that his prognosis is poor and that any effort invested in him is wasted. The psychiatrist, in particular, should study the patient and his interactions with staff, family, and friends to determine what elements are impeding the patient's motivation and what elements are beneficial to it [63].

Even though patients and staff actually belong to two different communities, there must be a common set of values applicable to both, or the unit cannot run efficiently. This requires that the patient accept certain ward rules—a minimum therapeutic package, so to speak. As a patient's definition of such a package inevitably will differ from the staff's definition, a balance in the scope of required values must be achieved. If the package is too restrictive and requires too much standardized behavior, the patient will not be able to agree to it. If, however, the package is too lenient and requires very little standardized behavior, then the unit may not function properly and the therapy may suffer.

Staff must, then, respect some of the freedoms of the patient, and they must give him areas of choice. One of the freedoms the patient must be allowed is the right to believe what he wishes so long as it does not conflict with the minimal therapeutic package. For instance, when a patient says, "I will walk again," staff must not intrude with their medical knowledge; they must permit the patient his belief. They must never try to convince the patient that, indeed, he will never walk again whatever his faith, even if they know that ambulation is impossible from a medical standpoint.

There is a therapeutic reason for noninterference that extends beyond the issue of the patient's freedom. Patients need to structure their recovery in their own ways except when it interferes with the functioning of the ward. Recognizing this need to structure one's own life, the professional can realize that what the patient says at one stage of his development may be said in an effort to cope with his debilitation. The professional can then help the patient to examine other possible alternatives. He might say, for example, "I can understand that you feel the possibility that you may walk again, but you should also consider the other possibility. You might permanently have less than full motion, and we must examine that alternative as well." This approach will extend the patient's range of possibilities without being intrusive and without limiting him to the professional's own conclusions about his condition.

The main consideration in socializing patients into the rehabilitation program is that the goal is socialization limited to a minimum therapeutic package, not socialization to a specific way of life. Staff must continually ask themselves, "Are we insisting on anything more than is necessary for meeting the therapeutic goals for the patient? Are we asking for more than a minimum package? Are we asking a patient, for instance, to eat breakfast every morning because we have decided that breakfast is good for him, even though there is no real evidence to show that breakfast has ever helped anyone?" If the demands made by staff come from personal conviction rather than from ward policy, staff are intruding on the patient's freedom and causing patient dissatisfaction.

Patients arrive on the ward with their own set of expectations, and this may fit more or less agreeably with the reality they encounter. Some expect the unit to be a very active place, functioning twenty-four hours a day; other expect to come for a rest and perhaps a few therapeutic exercises. Some patients come expecting a great deal of support; others enter expecting to be ignored or rejected because of their disability. Staff should attempt to discover early in the treatment what the patient's expectations are, always remembering, of course, that just as staff expectations change with experience, so will the patient's expectations evolve during his stay on the unit. The staff must learn initially what the patient expects from the ward, and then they should keep track of how those expectations change.

It is easy for a patient to isolate himself on a rehabilitation unit. The environment is such a change from anything he will have been accustomed to that unless a very strong effort is made by staff to create a sense of community among patients, patients will tend to avoid association with others on the unit and with the unit in general. Often, the patient who withdraws is fearful of losing something were he to accept contact, and it is the staff's job to find out what this something is. Frequently, the isolated patient is tacitly saying, "As long as I'm isolated, I'm not one of those people–I'm not one of the disabled. I'm going to stay right here, and I'll take care of myself." This is a common stance for a rehabilitation patient, and staff should respect the patient's feelings in the earlier stages of hospitalization. At the same time, staff should try to explore the patient's fears with him and try to understand what is causing them. Ultimately, staff should help the patient move outward to sample the environment and explore whether his fears are, in fact, reasonable.

If a patient insists on remaining isolated after an initial period of time has elapsed, then a staff person should be assigned to spend time with the patient, trying to keep his social awareness and skills alive much the same as he would exercise the patient's muscles. The patient must not be permitted to withdraw into himself where he might truly regress psychologically and then present an almost impossible problem for the staff.

As the loss of a part of one's function, a loss of ability, is a constant loss, staff must be prepared to accept the patient's grief as a continuing emotion. With the loss of a loved person, at some point one realizes the loss is forever and recovers. The loss of part of oneself is a daily loss–it confronts the person every hour of his existence. The patient must be allowed to grieve at the same time as he is being helped to adapt to his loss.

Patients' Psychosocial Needs

The unit we studied failed to meet the psychosocial needs of its rehabilitation patients. This occurred in part because the unit segmented the patient's care and in part because it denied or ignored the fact that the patient would have to face the community and find a place to live within it. Those responsible for the treatment program must learn to see rehabilitation as a long-term process, a process involving not only the hospital but the community. If people working on rehabilitation were to see their work as extending into society, they would have much more difficulty limiting their concern to the patient's progress while on the unit and ignoring his fate once he was discharged.

The future caregivers in the community should be integrated into the rehabilitation program so that they become involved with the patients whom they will later be helping to adjust to society, and there should be persons whose job it is to keep track of rehabilitation patients, making sure that no one is abandoned at any stage and that no one falls between the cracks of the system. Finally, at each stage of a patient's treatment, there should be an evaluation of the patient's social and psychological adaptation so that new areas can be explored to prepare for the patient's changing needs.

These recommendations may sound both idealistic and uneconomical, but from a cost-benefit point of view, society would be the winner. Analogous to the treatment of mental patients, rehabilitation treatment actually will save society money. Many people are upset because a patient has to pay approximately $2,500 for a year of psychotherapy, forgetting that were a patient to be hospitalized (at $200 a day), the same cost would be accrued in ten to twelve days, and the patient would not get the same benefits. The same can be said about rehabilitation care. It probably would be advantageous to pay for more consistent treatment than to pay for the acute care treatment problems that almost inevitably come up from time to time.

Support Systems

The peer or self-help group was a potential therapeutic resource the rehabilitation unit we studied did not utilize. There is no question that persons who have experienced the same problems as the patients could offer valuable aid on a rehabilitation unit. No one can understand another person, whether he be disabled, psychotic, or alcoholic, in the same way as someone who has had the same experience [64]. Even the most sensitive and sympathetic professional can understand only by analogy what the person who has had the same problem can know directly. Furthermore, a sense of mutual identification is possible among peers that no professional-client relationship can or should imitate.

A self-help group can serve many functions for rehabilitation patients. It can demonstrate to the patient how far he may be able to progress; veteran amputees, for instance, can dramatically illustrate to other amputees what adaptations are possible. A self-help group can also assist the patient in working out the psychosocial implications of his disability. It can make the individual feel more at liberty to express his problems, articulate his worries, anger, and sorrow because he is talking to people who will understand what he is feeling.

Despite the potentially positive contributions that peer or self-help groups can make, their assistance is not often requested. The staff often resist self-help groups because the group members usually possess a good deal of professional experience and some professional knowledge. As a result, the real professionals on a unit may feel uncomfortable with "semiprofessionals." They may fear that they will work against the staff rather than with them, or that they might raise objections to the staff's treatment performance. They may also fear that self-help groups would unite the patients against the staff. By no means unique to rehabilitation staff, this resistance can be seen in psychiatric institutions in relation to Recovery, Inc., and was once characteristic of alcoholic hospitals in their reaction to Alcoholics Anonymous.

Staff are not the only persons wary of self-help groups; often, the families of patients oppose any assistance from such groups. Afraid that the group will lower the patient's goals, that the patient will settle for being a partially recovered person rather than a "normal" human being, families often bitterly resent self-help groups because their goals for patients are limited. Families fear that contact with these groups will lower rather than elevate the patient's aspirations.

One person should be responsible for incorporating a self-help group's assistance into the therapy of the unit. He should act as the administrator and confront the anxieties of the staff and families. He should also serve as liaison among staff, family, and self-help group.

That families are both a potential source of support for patients and a potential problem has long been recognized. But the result of this awareness has usually been that the good is thrown away with the bad and that families are not used at all in a patient's rehabilitation treatment. We discussed briefly in Chapter 4 some of the reasons why families are not utilized in rehabilitation programs, and we would like here to recommend that closer examination be made of the family as a potentially positive resource. By evaluating the family, by analyzing its interaction with the patient, we can determine whether the particular family seems likely to be supportive or destructive. The decision about whether or not to use a family could then be made. Families must not be summarily rejected as sources of patient support; rather, staff must recognize both the pluses and the minuses of enlisting the family and decide on the merits of the individual case.

Budgeting

The economic limitations of the rehabilitation unit must be carefully considered in the planning stage [65]. Realistic boundaries must be recognized so that the integrity of the unit as a whole can be maintained, and estimates of the financial support needed and the financial support available must be made. Many long-term care units have run into problems because they overestimated the federal government's willingness to support patients in expensive care facilities. The core functions of the unit, the number of patients the unit will serve, the staffing needs, and the unit's finanacial relationship to the hospital community must all be considered in determining the unit's economic needs.

As there are limits to what society will be willing to give, estimates of income must be conservative. At the same time, however, it should be remembered that there will always be people who are injured or disabled as a result of illness, strokes, trauma, or industrial and other injuries. Society is also taking more responsibility for those injuries caused by use of insecticides, chemicals, and other pollutants. Society's greater awareness of its responsibility to its injured or maimed members can also be considered when planning a unit.

Community Considerations

The rehabilitation unit should be located in a place that makes sense for the community, much as an auditorium or a community college is situated where it will provide maximum service. The unit should be in a relatively attractive area, and it should be near a hospital where it will have available the required personnel and supplies.

Although medical organizations always resent external controls, particularly from nonspecialists, the community should play a role in determining the unit's criteria for admissions, duration of stay, and discharge [66]. Whatever the price paid in giving up complete control, the organization more than gains by the community's support and involvement. Because the community is one part of the voice of reality, that voice must be heard before it can be negotiated with. All communities have needs, and one of these needs is to know that it is doing good, that it is being charitable and delivering quality care. Fulfillment of this need is the community's reward for supporting a therapeutic unit, and thus both the medical unit and the community benefit from the relationship. Because the community must be satisfied if it is to continue its support, it is essential that the medical organization carefully assess where the needs of the community lie and how they can best be accommodated when the unit is in its planning stages.

Epilogue

All human beings are supported by ritual, and society has ceremonies to mark each change in a person's life. Birth, death, marriage, divorce, promotion, retirement—all have their accompanying rites, and we find that without ritual we can handle neither happy nor unhappy transitions comfortably.

So, too, with organizations. Military services have rituals for change of command; governmental bodies have highly stylized ceremonies for shifting power; and religious organizations are perhaps the most deeply ingrained in ritual of any group. As individuals are troubled without the guidance of ritual, when an organization has no prescribed procedure for meeting a change it manages that change only uneasily. This discomfort was evident in the phasing out of the rehabilitation unit. We have no ceremony to smooth over or depersonalize such an ending, just as we have no ceremony for firing a worker. Although hospital units may be expanded or contracted according to the needs of the organization, the closing of a unit is an infrequent event. We are unprepared for infrequent events.

This unit had been inaugurated with some fanfare. There was an open house and a tour, and the ward was displayed with pride to the faculty and staff of the hospital and to relatives of staff members. Its demise was marked only by a few private wakes. There was an element of embarrassment. Those outside of the unit hoped that memories of it would fade quickly and, in fact, they did.

Those who worked on the ward were touched by what they saw as the unit's failure. They were persons who wanted to be winners, not losers. They wanted to be thought of as winners, associated with winning organizations. They saw their association with a losing enterprise as a reflection on them and feared that others would judge them as incompetent because they were associated with a failure. They judged themselves as unlucky, and they feared that others would shun them because of the danger in associating with unlucky people. Fortunately, there were some few outsiders who understood the impact on the leadership and staff of the unit and attempted to limit the trauma and initiate the healing process.

This book has attempted to look beyond any individual flaws or faults and to see the problems this unit faced in larger, more systematic terms. We feel strongly that only by depersonalizing the events and circumstances that lead to success or failure can we begin to understand the elements that contribute not only to the failure of this particular unit or the psychiatric unit before it but also to the success or failure of any comparable program. In effect, we have tried to ritualize, to depersonalize, the transitions this unit experienced and to focus on what it might have in common with other potential units rather than on its unique problems. The value of ceremony is that it intensifies the universal while deemphasizing the individual, so we can find what is personal to us in what is common to all. We have applied this same value to the study of the rehabilitation unit in the hope that our recommendations can serve as a guide, so that other units may prevent or at least anticipate some of the problems that proved fatal for the program of this study.

References

1. Brodsky, C.M. The culture of the small psychiatric unit in a general hospital. *American Journal of Psychotherapy*, 25:246-57, 1970.

2. Davis, F. Deviance disavowal: The management of strained interaction by the visibly handicapped. *Social Problems*, 9:121-32, 1961.

3. Silverman, S. *Psychological Aspects of Physical Symptoms: A Dynamic Study of Forty-five Hospitalized Medical Patients*. New York: Appleton-Century-Crofts, 1968.

4. Frank, J.D. Psychotherapy of bodily disease: An overview. *Psychotherapy and Psychosomatics*, 26:192-202, 1975.

5. Lipowski, Z.J. Psychosocial aspects of disease. *Annals of Internal Medicine*, 71:1197-1206, 1969.

6. Lipowski, Z.J. Psychiatry of somatic diseases: Epidemiology, pathogenesis, classification. *Comprehensive Psychiatry*, 16:105-24, 1975.

7. Kutner, B. Rehabilitation: Whose goals? Whose priorities? *Archives of Physical Medicine and Rehabilitation*, 52:284-87, 1971.

8. Herrerin, E.A., Katz, A.H. Issues and orientations in the evaluation of rehabilitation programs. A review article. *Rehabilitation Literature*, 32:66-74, 1971.

9. French, J.R.P. Person role fit. *Occupation and Mental Health*, 3:15-20, 1973.

10. Insel, P.M., Moos, R.H. The social environment. In P.M. Insel and R.H. Moos (eds.), *Health and the Social Environment*. Lexington, MA: D.C. Heath, 1974.

11. Price, R.H. Etiology, the social environment, and the prevention of psychological difficulties. In P.M. Insel and R.H. Moos (eds.), *Health and the Social Environment*. Lexington, MA: D.C. Heath, 1974.

12. Beers, M., Huse, E.F. A systems approach to organization development. *Journal of Applied Behavioral Science*, 8:79-101, 1972.

13. Caplan, G. *Support Systems and Community Mental Health. Lectures on Concept Development*. New York: Behavioral Publications, 1974.

14. Moos, R.H. *The Human Context: Environmental Determinants of Behavior*. New York: Wiley, 1976.

15. Moos, R.H., Smail, P. Characterizing treatment environments. In R.H. Moos (ed.), *Evaluating Treatment Environments; A Social Ecological Approach*. New York: Wiley, 1974.

16. Anderson, S.E., Good, L.R., Hurtig, W.E. Designing a mental health center to replace a county hospital. *Hospital and Community Psychiatry*, 27: 807-13, 1976.

17. Erickson, E.R. Be bold or fold. Converting a chronic disease hospital to a physical rehabilitation center. *Hospital Forum*, 14:7-8, 27-28, 1971.

18. Berkovitz, M., Johnson, W.G. Towards an economics of disability: The magnitude and structural transfer of medical costs. *The Journal of Human Resources*, 5:271-97, 1970.

19. Wilson, R.N. The social structure of a general hospital. In J.K. Skipper and R.L. Leonard (eds.), *Social Interaction and Patient Care*. Philadelphia: Lippincott, 1965.

20. Skipper, J.K., Leonard, R.L. The importance of communication. In J.K. Skipper and R.L. Leonard (eds.), *Social Interaction and Patient Care*. Philadelphia: Lippincott, 1965.

21. Goldberg, D. Principles of rehabilitation. *Comprehensive Psychiatry*, 15:237-48, 1974.

22. Menninger, K.A. Psychiatric aspects of physical disability. In J.F. Garrett (ed.), *Psychological Aspects of Physical Disability* (Rehabilitation Service Series No. 310). Washington, D.C.: Office of Vocational Rehabilitation, DHEW, 1953.

23. Weinstein, M.R. The illness process: Psychosocial hazards of disability programs. *J.A.M.A.*, 204:209-15, 1968.

24. Blum, L.H. *Reading between the Lines: Doctor-Patient Communication*. New York: International Universities Press, 1972.

25. Berger, S. Paraplegia. In J.F. Garrett (ed.), *Psychological Aspects of Physical Disability* (Rehabilitation Service Series No. 310). Washington, D.C.: Office of Vocational Rehabilitation, DHEW, 1953.

26. Becker, M.C., Abrams, K.S., Onder, J. Goal setting: A joint patient-staff method. *Archives of Physical Medicine and Rehabilitation*, 55:87-89, 1974.

27. Levinson, H. *Organizational Diagnosis*. Cambridge, MA: Harvard University Press, 1972.

28. Stanton, A., Schwartz, M. *The Mental Hospital*. New York: Basic Books, 1954.

29. English, H.B., English, A.C. *A Comprehensive Dictionary of Psychological and Psychoanalytic Terms*. London: Longmans, Green, 1958.

30. Berne, E. *Games People Play: The Psychology of Human Relationships*. New York: Grove Press, 1964.

31. Engel, G.L. A life setting conducive to illness: The giving-up—given-up complex. *Annals of Internal Medicine*, 69:293-300, 1968.

32. Shontz, F.C. Severe chronic illness. In S.L. Garrett and E. Levine (eds.), *Psychological Practices with the Physically Disabled*. New York: Columbia University Press, 1962.

33. Bellak, L. *Psychology of Physical Illness. Psychiatry Applied to Medicine, Surgery, and the Specialties*. New York: Grune and Stratton, 1952.

34. Starkey, P.D. Sick-role retention as a factor in nonrehabilitation. *Journal of Counseling Psychology*, 15:75-9, 1967.

35. Wright, B. *Physical Disability: A Psychological Approach*. New York: Harper, 1960.

36. Barker, R.G., Wright, B.A., Gonick, M.R. *Adjustment to Physical Handicap and Illness: A Survey of the Social Psychology of Physique and Disability*. New York: Social Science Research Council, 1946.

37. Waitzkin, H. Latent functions of the sick role in various institutional settings. *Social Science and Medicine*, 5:45-75, 1971.

38. Barker, R.G., Wright, B.A. The social psychology of adjustment to physical disability. In J.F. Garrett (ed.), *Psychological Aspects of Physical Disability* (Rehabilitation Service Series No. 310). Washington, D.C.: Office of Vocational Rehabilitation, DHEW, 1953.

39. Rae, J.W. Rehabilitation: Today's responsibilities and challenges. *Archives of Physical Medicine and Rehabilitation*, 54:605-607, 1973.

40. Parsons, T. *The Social System*. Glencoe, IL: The Free Press, 1951.

41. Ling, T.M. Psychological and occupational effects of illness and accident. In T.M. Ling (ed.), *Mental Health and Human Relations in Industry*. London: H.K. Lewis, 1954.

42. McDaniel, J.W. *Physical Disability and Human Behavior*. New York: Pergamon Press, 1969.

43. Kerr, N. Staff expectations for disabled persons: Helpful or harmful. *Rehabilitation Counseling Bulletin*, 14:85-94, 1970.

44. Nathanson, M., Bergman, P.S., Gordon, G.G. Denial of illness: Its occurrence in one hundred consecutive cases of hemiplegia. *Archives of Neurology and Psychiatry*, 68:380-87, 1952.

45. Kerr, N. Understanding the process of adjustment to disability. *Journal of Rehabilitation*, 27:16-18, 1961.

46. Howard, J. Humanization and dehumanization of health care. In J. Howard and A. Strauss (eds.), *Humanizing Health Care*. New York: Wiley, 1975.

47. Schlesinger, L.E. Staff authority and patient participation in rehabilitation. *Rehabilitation Literature*, 24:247-49, 1965.

48. Kutner, B. Professional antitherapy. *Journal of Rehabilitation*, 35: 16-18, 1969.

49. Kingdon, D.R. *Matrix Organization: Managing Information Technologies*. New York: Barnes and Noble, 1973.

50. Wedel, K.R. Matrix design for human service organizations. *Administration in Mental Health*, Fall, 1976.

51. French, J.R.P. The social environment and mental health. *Journal of Social Issues*, 19:39-56, 1963.

52. Kiritz, S., Moos, R.H. Physiological effects of social environments. *Psychosomatic Medicine*, 36:96-114, 1974.

53. Cleland, D.E., King, W.R. *Systems Analysis and Project Management*. New York: McGraw-Hill, 1968.

54. Bennett, A.C. A checklist for identifying areas of improvement. *Hospital Topics*, 52:6, 8, 1974.

55. Kennedy, O.G., Hamilton, B.B., Galliers, J. A conceptual model for planning the delivery of rehabilitation services. *Archives of Physical Medicine and Rehabilitation*, 53:461-69, 1972.

56. Neuhauser, D. The hospital as a matrix organization. *Hospital Administration*, 17:8-25, 1972.

57. Stang, L., Sprague, J.B., Holley, L.S. Implementation of rehabilitation services in community hospitals. *American Journal of Public Health*, 64:1081-88, 1974.

58. Le Compte, W.F. The taxonomy of a treatment environment. *Archives of Physical Medicine and Rehabilitation*, 53:109-14, 1972.

59. Vineberg, S.E. The environment as a network of judgments regarding staff roles. *Archives of Physical Medicine and Rehabilitation*, 53:102-108, 1972.

60. Haney, W.V. *Communication and Organizational Behavior*. Homewood, IL: Irwin, 1973.

61. Abramson, A.S., Kutner, B. A Bill of Rights for the Disabled (Editorial). *Archives of Physical Medicine and Rehabilitation*, 53:99-100, 1972.

62. Anderson, T.P. An alternative frame of reference for rehabilitation: The helping process versus the medical model. *Archives of Physical Medicine and Rehabilitation*, 56:101-104, 1975.

63. Lomos, P. Family interaction and the sick role. In J.O. Wisdom and H.H. Wolff (eds.), *The Role of Psychosomatic Disorder in Adult Life*. Proceedings of the Society for Psychosomatic Research at the Royal College of Physicians at London, November, 1961.

64. Dembo, T. The utilization of psychological knowledge in rehabilitation. In J. Stubbins (ed.), *Social and Psychological Aspects of Disability. A Handbook for Practitioners*. Baltimore, MD: University Park Press, 1977.

65. Ewell, C.M., Jr., Johnson, A.C., Von Ehren, W.R. Administrators identify the problems. *Hospitals*, 48:52-5, 1974.

66. Hightower, M.D. Rehabilitation: A part of the community or apart from the community. *American Journal of Occupational Therapy*, 28:296-98, 1974.

Index

About the Authors

Carroll M. Brodsky is a professor of psychiatry at the University of California School of Medicine in San Francisco. He founded and directs the Work Clinic at the University of California, a project that has received national recognition. In addition, he serves as a consultant to the California Workers' Compensation Institute and to the Nevada Industrial Commission.

Dr. Brodsky received the Ph.D. in anthropology from Catholic University in Washington, D.C., and the M.D. from the University of California School of Medicine in San Francisco. He was responsible for psychiatric liaison and consultation to the rehabilitation unit that is the subject of this book.

Robert T. Platt is an assistant clinical professor of psychiatry at the University of California School of Medicine in San Francisco. He was a consultant to the rehabilitation unit described in this book, and is a faculty member of the Work Clinic at the University of California. He is a graduate of the University of Michigan and received his medical education at the State University of New York, Downstate Medical Center, Brooklyn, New York. He did his residency in psychiatry at the Langley Porter Neuropsychiatric Institute, under the auspices of the National Institute of Mental Health. He consults with agencies and organizations in problems of diagnosing and treating disabled persons.

RC
439
.B84

1978